PALS Provider Manual

Pediatric Advanced Life Support

Jane John-Nwankwo   RN, MSN

PALS PROVIDER MANUAL:
Pediatric Advanced Life Support

Copyright © 2015 by Jane John-Nwankwo RN, MSN

All rights reserved. No part of this book may be reproduced or transmitted in any form or by any means without written permission from the author.

ISBN-13: 978-1511533942

ISBN-10: 1511533943

Printed in the United States of America.

Dedication

To all who love to save tiny, but BIG lives

OTHER TITLES FROM THE SAME AUTHOR:

1. Work At Home Jobs For Nurses & Other Healthcare Professionals
2. Nurses' Romance Series
3. Hightime you made a move! An inspirational and motivational book
4. Patient Care Technician Exam Review Questions: PCT Test Prep
5. Weight Loss Inspiration
6. EKG Technician Study Guide
7. BLS for Healthcare Providers Student Manual
8. Phlebotomy Test Prep Vol 1, 2, & 3
9. It's in Your Hands: Five Strategies to Achieving Your Life Dreams
10. How to make a million in nursing

And Many More Books

Visit www.janejohn-nwankwo.com

What you will learn

- Team Resuscitation Concepts
- What Actually Happens in Mega Codes
- BLS & PALS Surveys
- Pediatric Assessment
- Acute Coronary Syndrome Management
- Stroke Management
- Recognition of Basic Dysrhythmias
- Plus 160 Review Questions

Section 1

PALS stands for Pediatric Advanced Life Support. It is simply the part two of Basic Life Support (BLS) for pediatrics. It is a training offered to healthcare providers to provide emergency cardiovascular life support and administer the tools to effectively treat emergencies in pediatrics. After studying this manual, healthcare providers should feel comfortable and familiar with the following topics:

- Effective resuscitation team dynamics
- Pediatric Assessment
- BLS Survey(systematic CABD approach)
- PALS Survey(systematic ABCD approach), including situational algorithms
- Pathophysiology of some critical conditions
- Identifying and treating medical conditions that put patients at risk for cardiac arrest

Pediatric Assessment (level of consciousness, breathing, color)

Precise assessment of a child with an acute illness or suffering from an injury requires certain crucial knowledge and skills. Most of the children presenting in the ER often have a mild, moderate illness and injury and stay alert. In the assessment of these patients' illnesses and injuries, several methodologies and severity scales can be incorporated for assessing the levels of consciousness. However, these methodologies often lack accuracy, especially when it comes to infants and toddlers (Donnelly, 2009). This implies that although the methods will help in classifying the moderate to critically ill or injured child, it will however not help in the recognition of crucial signs that help in noting the early symptoms of system strain in the sick or wounded child who is still operating well or looks well. A nurse needs to apply critical thinking in assessing pediatrics as their shift from consciousness to unconsciousness is very rapid.

1. **Evaluation-primary assessment, secondary assessment, diagnostic tests**

Diagnostic tests refer to any test that is used to determine the existence of an illness or disease. For example, there are cases where the test is carried out in order to fully diagnose someone or to affirm that a patient is free of any disease. Diagnostic tests include CT scans, bronchoscopy, x-rays, oesophageal ultrasound and angiography.

The main aim of carrying out primary assessment is to immediately identify life threatening problems. The primary assessment mainly aims at stabilizing the patient, identify life-threatening conditions in the patient in order of risk and initiate for treatment immediately. Secondary assessment will come after the primary assessment has been fully carried out and the patient's vital signs have all been assessed. It comprises of checking the patient history and physical examination of the patient.

2. **Respiratory Assessment, Circulatory Assessment**

Respiratory assessment consists of four main components, which include inspection, palpation, percussion and auscultation. Inspection involves the medical practitioner using their eyes and ears to assess a varying number of things about their patients. Some of the main things that should be observed include pursed lip breathing, noisy breathing, skin color, coughing, respiratory rate, patterns, and chest wall abnormalities.

In the palpation phase, the healthcare personnel uses their fingers and hands during the physical examination. They will touch and feel the patient's body in order to determine the consistency, size, texture, tenderness and location of a body organ or body part. Percussion on the other hand involves the technique of tapping body hands by using the fingers and certain instruments during the physical examination. It is often used to determine the presence or absence of fluids in certain body organs and the borders, size and consistency of body organs (Baren, 2008).

Percussion of a body organ normally produces a certain sound that will in turn indicate the presence of a certain tissue within that particular body part or organ. Lastly, there is auscultation. During auscultation, the patient is supposed to sit upright while taking in deep breaths through the mouth. Any outside noise should be eliminated if possible. The examiner will then listen to the sounds arising within the body organs.

While assessing circulation, the medical practitioner should determine whether the child has a pulse or is in shock. One should keep in mind that children and infants are only capable of tolerating only small amounts of blood loss before they suffer circulatory compromise. It is important to assess and control any bleeding early in the circulatory assessment. Circulatory assessment should not only focus on the circulatory status but also try to correct any inadequate circulation to other body organs of the infant or child. The main measures of circulatory assessment are heart rate and blood pressure. However, changes in the skin percussion can be used as indicators of compensated shock.

Types of shock: (Hypovolemic, distributive, cardiogenic, obstructive)

a. *Cardiogenic Shock*

In cardiogenic shock, the forward flow of blood is often inadequate due to a defect in the cardiac function. It normally happens when the heart cannot properly pump blood through the body system. This could be due to impairment caused to the heart from myocardial infarction that results in enough damage to the heart to impair its proper functioning. Furthermore, a disease or virus could also be a cause of cardiogenic shock.

b. *Hypovolemic Shock*

Hypo simply means lack of or low, while volemic refers to fluid volume. In an instance when a patient is injured and profusely bleeding, the volume of blood that the body is able to deliver reduces substantially resulting to the patient experiencing hypovolemic shock. This kind of shock is quite common in patients who have suffered from trauma and have external bleeding. However, a patient can equally suffer from internal bleeding from an illness or injury, which can quickly result in the patient falling into a hypovolemic shock state.

c. *Distributive Shock*

Distributive shock occurs when the intravascular volume is markedly abnormal due to a decrease in vascular resistance, such as it happens to occur in fainting where blood pools in the venous instead of the arterial portion of the blood flow.

Cardiac output may be augmented, normal or small in patients who experience distributive shock. Several causes may cause distributive shock such as septic shock, neurogenic shock, anaphylactic shock and acute adrenal insufficiency. However, there are drugs that result in vasodilation thus resulting in the patient experiencing distributive shock (Baren, 2008).

d. *Obstructive Shock*

The main characteristic of obstructive shock is the impedance of sufficient cardiac filling of the ventricles leading to a significant decrease in the cardiac output. As the distribution of blood decreases, the patients' tissues may begin to die because of lack of oxygen and necessary nutrients. There are certain patients who have a high risk of suffering from obstructive shock such as those on bed rest and those who have mobility issues and do not move around so much. Furthermore, patients with chest injuries have a higher risk of suffering from obstructive shock.

Diagnostic tests: Arterial blood gas

Arterial blood gas is the measurement of the oxygen level in the blood flowing through the arteries. The process normally involves puncturing an artery with a thin needle and drawing a small amount blood from the artery. The most commonly chosen puncture for this process is the radial artery.

The main reason for carrying out this test is in order to determine the blood pH level, the part pressure of carbon dioxide and oxygen and the level of bicarbonate in the blood. In addition, there are instances where the test determines the lactate level. However, the required sample to carry out the arterial blood gas test may be difficult to acquire because of the diminished pulses in some patients and constant patient movement (King, 2008).

Diminished pulses may be a reflection of low blood pressure or poor peripheral circulation in the patient as a result of the illness. The constant movement is due to the pain that comes as a result of the arterial puncture. In an infant who weighs less than 30 pounds, arterial blood can be obtained from the capillary stick instead, and in the case of a newborn, it is obtained from the umbilical catheter. Although arterial puncture is a skill that can easily be learned, there may be instances where certain complications may come about as a result. Such complications include trauma and occlusion, infection, vessel spasm and embolization. However, in a case where a skilled practitioner performs arterial puncture, it offers safe and reliable information, which is useful in patient management.

Venous Blood Gas

Venous blood gas (VBG) is a substitute method used in the measurement or estimation of carbon dioxide and pH in the blood that does not require arterial puncture.

VBG is most preferred as compared to ABG, particularly for patients in the intensive care unit given that they already have a central venous catheter from which the venous blood can easily be obtained.

The VBG test is useful in assessing oxygen and carbon dioxide gas exchange, respiratory functions such as hypoxia and acid/base balance in the patients. Furthermore, it can also be incorporated in the evaluation of asthma, chronic obstructive pulmonary disease and various types of lung disease such as coronary artery disease. Abnormal results of the VBG tests may be due to metabolic, lung and kidney diseases. However, patients who may have a history of head or neck injuries will also likely have abnormal VBG results (Donnelly, 2009)

Hemoglobin and Hematocrit

Both the hemoglobin and the hematocrit refer to specific characteristics of the red blood cells, but they however measure different things. The hemoglobin is a compound in the red blood cells that transports oxygen to other cells in the body. The hemoglobin tests measures how much hemoglobin is present in the blood. The test is often carried out when doctors want to determine the patient's general health and patients' blood chemistry. The hematocrit test on the other hand is carried out to determine the total percentage of the volume of the blood that contains the red blood cells. The measurement will be dependent on the number of the red blood cells and the size of the red blood cells.

Central venous pressure monitoring

The central venous pressure (CVP) is the direct measurement of blood pressure in the central veins adjacent to the heart. It shows the average right atrial pressure and are most of the times used to estimate the right ventricular preload. Although the CVP does not measure the blood volume directly, it may however be used from time to time. In CVP monitoring, a catheter is inserted through a vein and advanced until the tip lies in or on the right atrium. Given the fact that there are no valves present between the junction of the vena cava and the right atrium, the pressure reading at the end of the diastole directly transfers to the catheter. CVP monitoring is important because it gives the necessary information pertaining to the body's blood volume or fluid status and the right ventricular function. CVP can be monitored intermittently or continuously. There are three main approaches used in the measuring of the pressure in the right atrium. One would be using a water manometer attached to the attached to the CV catheter. Second would be using a line placed directly into the right atrium which is then attached to the transducer system. Lastly, would be using a proximal lumen of a pulmonary artery catheter.

The normal CVP ranges from 5 to 10 cm H_2O. A number of underlying conditions that may alter venous return, flowing blood volume or cardiac activity may in turn impact on the CVP. For instance, if the circulating blood was to increase due to increase in venous return to the heart, the CVP is most likely to rise. On the other hand, if the flowing volume decreases, the CVP will drop. Overdistention or underfilling of the venous collecting system can easily be identified by monitoring the CVP before the clinical symptoms become apparent. The CVP can be measures in instances where the patients with hypertension are not responding to the basic clinical management implemented, or in patients requiring infusions or inotropes, or in patients who seem to be experiencing continuing hypervolemia secondary to major fluid loss or shifts (Parthasarathy, 2013).

Invasive Arterial pressure monitoring

Invasive blood pressure (IBP) monitoring is a commonly employed method in the Intensive Care Unit (ICU) and in the operating room. It entails the insertion of a catheter into a suitable artery and displaying the recorded pressure wave on the monitor. Patients who are undergoing invasive blood pressure monitoring should be under close supervision constantly given that they may likely suffer blood loss in any case the line comes off. The method is often reserved for critically ill patients who are likely to experience rapid changes in their blood pressure.

Normal or acceptable blood pressure varies from one patient to another depending on the patient's age, health status and clinical information. At birth, the expected blood pressure is normally 80 mmHg. This number rises steadily through childhood, such that in a young adult the expected blood pressure is 100/80 mmHg. In order to determine whether the recorded reading is normal for that particular patient, it shall be compared to the "normal" for that patient. In the incorporation of this technique in blood measurement, the cannula is place into an artery (normally radial, dorsalis pedis or brachial). The cannula will then be connected to a sterile system filled with fluid which is then connected to an electronic patient monitor. The main benefit of this method is that the pressure is measured beat-by-beat and the waveform easily readable and displayed for monitoring.

Chest x-ray, echocardiogram, peak expiratory flow rate

Peak flow rate is a simple, quantitative, reproducible measurement of the existence and severity of air flow obstruction. It is an important tool often used in the monitoring, exacerbations and daily long term monitoring. Peak expiratory flow (PEF) can be measured by the use of Mini Wright peak flow meters which are inexpensive and affordable to many. PEF is a quick and easy way for health care practitioners to measure and record predicted normal PEF values, while taking into consideration the height and age of the child as a point of reference.

However, the value which is considered "normal" is of a rather wide range and hence the test is dependent on the effort of the pediatrician. Health care practitioners can easily teach their patients to carry the PEF test on their own given the easy nature of the method.

Respiratory distress and failure

Respiratory distress is a state of increased work of breathing, while respiratory failure is a state inadequate oxygenation or ventilation. Respiratory failure may or may not be preceded by respiratory failure. Assessment of an infant's respiratory status often begins with the Pediatric Assessment Triangle. Infants and children often have unique clinical condition that may result in respiratory problems. Respiratory distress is a form of respiratory failure that comes about as a result of varying disorders that may cause fluid to accumulate in the lungs and low oxygen levels in the blood. According to research, quick identification of respiratory distress in in the pediatric patient is crucial before it escalates into respiratory failure. The main symptoms of respiratory failure often manifest themselves in the patient 24 to 48 hours after injury, but may take up to 5 days to be notable in the patient. The patient is likely to have shortness of breath, and usually shallow and rapid breathing. Crackling or wheezing sounds can be heard when the pediatrician auscultates the lungs. The small oxygen availability in the blood will also cause the child's skin to be cyanotic.

Conversely, respiratory failure is a situation in which one or all the gas exchange functions fails i.e. oxygenation and carbon dioxide elimination. The situation can either be acute or chronic. It is safe to construe that this condition will likely occur in a patient whose respiratory distress was not handled properly. The main difference between respiratory distress and respiratory failure is that in respiratory distress the patent is still breathing, while in respiratory failure the patient stops breathing completely (Taussig, 2008). Respiratory failure normally occurs when the patients' lungs are incapable of properly removing carbon dioxide from the infant's blood. This will in turn result in too much accumulation of carbon dioxide in the system which will harm the patient's body organs. There are certain illnesses that that affect infants breathing that will result in respiratory failure such as chronic obstructive pulmonary disease (prevents air from properly flowing in and out of the system) and spinal cord injuries (may damage nerves that control breathing).

Management of upper respiratory airway obstruction

The most shared cause of upper respiratory obstruction is the tongue. The management of a patient with upper respiratory obstruction will vary depending on the cause of the obstruction, the level of skill and competence of the rescuer, and the availability of aids to perform the necessary airway techniques.

Obstruction of the upper airway is a life threatening condition that if not properly managed may possibly result in the patient's death. The main aim is to secure the patient from getting a heart attack or possibly suffering irreversible brain damage that can take place within minutes of the airway obstruction..

Management of Lower respiratory Airway obstruction.

Lower respiratory airway obstruction normally results from the infection or irritation from certain particular particles or substances. It normally occurs between the larynx and the narrow passages of the lungs. The main symptoms include air trapping, an increased AP diameter and barrel chest. The common simple ways of helping a patient with lower airway obstruction include chin lift, jaw thrust and performing adjuncts.

Intraosseous access.

In a critical resuscitation circumstance, after the airway has been secured and adequate breathing and gas exchange fully established back to normal, the next priority should be to obtain vascular access. Most of the times, this is difficult to attain especially in children and infants. The physiologic progressions of shock and hypothermia with subsequent vascular tightening which are normally notable in the resuscitative state may later on complicate the issue of venous access and make it worse.

In addition, the expertise of most healthcare personnels when it comes to attending to children widely varies.

Instraosseous access has been used for years and is considered safe, reliable and can easily used by medical practitioners who are not highly skilled when it comes to handling children as a way of introducing blood products, colloids, medications and crystalloids into the regular circulation (Parthasarathy, 2013).

References

Baren, J. M. (2008). *Pediatric emergency medicine*. Philadelphia: Saunders/Elsevier.

Donnelly, L. F. (2009). *Fundamentals of pediatric radiology*. Philadelphia: Saunders.

Parthasarathy, A. (2013). *Partha's fundamentals of pediatrics*. New Delhi: Jaypee Brothers Publishers.

King, C., & Henretig, F. M. (2008). *Textbook of pediatric emergency procedures*. Philadelphia: Wolters Kluwer Health/Lippincott Williams & Wilkins.

Taussig, L. M., Landau, L. I., & Le, S. P. N. (2008). *Pediatric respiratory medicine*. Philadelphia: Mosby/Elsevier.

Resuscitation Teams

Resuscitation teams always arise when there is a code blue situation, or an individual's life is at stake. The Keys to successful medical teams are communication, teamwork and respect. Resuscitation team members must be able to communicate and interact with each other in a cohesive way, so as to increase chances of a successful resuscitation. The basis of a successful and efficient resuscitation team is the mastery of BLS and PALS skills and maintaining a professional and respectful relationship with each other and familiar with the various team roles. Specific roles of team leaders and members, and their interactions are discussed in more detail below.

Team Leaders usually assume the commanding role in resuscitation team, organizing and integrating members and their respective roles. A leader needs to be experienced in all areas of resuscitation. They should feel comfortable and competent to provide comprehensive care. They are there to lead team members through resuscitation efforts. The effective team leader is one that members feel at ease with.

Team members may not be experts at all tasks but must have vast experience at their assigned roles. They are responsible for knowing their task and the other members' task. Team members consists of:

-The time keeper

-The chest compressor

-The recorder

-The medication or IV nurse, etc.

Team members should be familiar and comfortable with the PALS algorithms. For the team to succeed, it is vital that all members are committed to the team and the patient's care at all times. Maintaining a respectful environment among all members will aid the success of resuscitation attempts.

Team interaction is based on solid communication, defined roles, awareness of members' stress and weaknesses, respect, and knowledge sharing. Each factor plays an integral part in successful resuscitation.

Communication Feedback and Acknowledgement

It is important to confirm that an order or course of action has been heard, interpreted and implemented as intended. Team members should clearly acknowledge the receipt of a message by providing eye contact and verbal confirmation. Once a task has been completed, members should verbally notify the team leader and wait for the next assignment. An effective team leader would then repeat received message from team member and, after confirming the task is completed, provide instructions for the next task. Moving on to implement another task while one is not completed can reduce the effectiveness of resuscitation. Quality patient care is the highest priority and this should be the teams' main focus.

Communicate Clearly & Effectively

Effective and clear team communication is vital to successful resuscitation. Deliver concise messages in a calm and straightforward manner. To reduce confusion, only one person should be speaking at a time. If a message was not clearly understood, members should ask for it to be repeated. Then, confirm what they heard by reiterating message to sender.

Define Roles and Acknowledge Personal Limitations

Defining individuals' roles is important so that tasks are not duplicated, missed or performed inadequately. Team leaders will assign roles to each member and each member should, in turn, accept only roles that they feel comfortable completing. Members should not work outside their skill level; someone should notify the team leader if they have been assigned a role that is outside their competency levels. If team members do find themselves in an unknown territory or situation, they should ask for help sooner rather than later. This is a team and each member is here to help. Tasks should be assigned evenly and appropriately to each available team member to ensure the most efficient care is provided.

Share Knowledge

To provide the best care to the patient, all team members should utilize shared knowledge. Shared information, possible treatment techniques or courses of action will enable the team to progress quickly and effectively. Team leaders should reinforce a sharing environment by asking members' suggestions, ideas or identification of overlooked diagnosis or treatment options.

When a task is completed incorrectly, team members are encouraged to offer their opinion or question the actions of another team member. When providing constructive criticism or alternative treatment methods, do so in a supporting, non-confrontational manner.

Analyze Resuscitation Efforts

Assessment of patient's status needs to be completed throughout resuscitation. Team members discuss next treatment steps and should be prepared to change treatment plan if necessary, effective team leader will review the resuscitation effort load and act within capacity of the team. Keeping a log of patient's progress and response to drugs will be helpful for a complete analysis.

BLS Survey

The BLS survey is a systematic approach to basic life support that any trained healthcare provider performs. This approach stresses early CPR and early defibrillation. It does not include advance interventions, such as advance airway techniques or drug administration. By using the BLS survey healthcare providers may achieve their goal of supporting or restoring effective oxygen ventilation, and circulation until ROSC (Return of Spontaneous Circulation) or initiation of ACLS or PALS interventions. Performing the action, the BLS survey substantially improves the patient's chance of survival and a good neurologic output.

Before conducting the BLS or PALS survey, look to make sure the scene is safe for you and the victim. This is because, for example if the case was an attempted murder, the murderer would not want the individual coming back to life, and so may return to finish the job and your life may not be spared either.

The BLS Survey uses a series of 4 sequential assessment steps designated by the numbers 1, 2, 3, and 4. Simultaneously with each assessment step, you should perform the appropriate corrective action before proceeding to the next step. Assessment is a key component in this approach (e.g. check pulse before starting chest compressions or attaching an AED). CABD stands for Compressions, Airway, Breathing & Defibrillation.

Remember **ASSESS** then **PERFORM** appropriate action.

1. **Check responsiveness-**

    - Tap and shout, "Are you all right?"
    - Check for an absent or abnormal breathing by looking at or scanning the chest for movement(not more than 10 seconds)

2. **Activate the emergency response system/ get AED (Automated External Defibrillator)**

3. **Circulation-**

    - Check the carotid pulse for 5 to 10 seconds

- If no pulse within 10 seconds, start CPR(30:2) beginning with chest compressions
- Switch providers every 2 minutes to avoid fatigue
- Avoid excessive ventilation
- If there is a pulse, start rescue breathing at 1 breathe every 5 to 6 seconds (10 to 12 breaths/ minute). Check pulse every 2 minutes

4. **Defibrillation-**
    - If no pulse, check for a shockable rhythm with an AED/ defibrillator as soon as it arrives
    - Provide shocks as indicated
    - Follow each shock immediately with CPR, beginning with compressions

Tips: The BLS survey no longer consists of the sequence "look, listen and feel" followed by 2 regular breaths. In essence, you still 'look, listen and feel' but very rapidly because it was discovered that healthcare providers continued to 'LOOK, LISTEN & FEEL' while the patient's chances of survival decreased. That is why the emphasis is to check for responsiveness and pulse for not more than 10 seconds. So, if you don't feel a pulse or are not sure if you feel a pulse, START COMPRESSIONS!

Assess		Action
Airway	Is the patient's airway open?	Open airway using noninvasive techniques such as head tilt chin lift or jaw thrust
Breathing	Is the patient breathing? Are the patient's respirations adequate?	Give 2 rescue breaths, each one lasting one second. Make sure the chest rises. Maintain a moderate ventilation rate and volume
Circulation	Does the patient have a pulse?	Check carotid pulse for 5-10 sec. Perform CPR until AED is available
Defibrillation	If there is not a pulse, check patient for a shockable rhythm using manual defibrillator or AED	Provide necessary shock. Immediately after shock, begin CPR start with chest compressions

PALS Survey

Pediatric Advanced life support (PALS) is an extension of BLS and is performed when the basic life support interventions have failed and advanced measures are needed. PALS is a set of clinical interventions for the urgent treatment of cardiac arrest and other life- threatening medical emergencies. It also refers to the knowledge and skills to deploy those interventions.

It often starts with analyzing a patient's heart rhythm with a manual defibrillator. In contrast to in the BLS, where the machine decides when and how to shock a patient the PALS team leader makes those decisions based on rhythms on the monitor and patients vital signs. The next step in PALS is insertion of intravenous (IV) lines and placement of various airway devices. Commonly used drugs, such as epinephrine, atropine and amiodarone, are then administered. At this time, the healthcare provider quickly searches for possible cause of cardiac arrest (i.e. heart attack, overdose, and trauma). Based on their diagnosis, more specific treatments are given. These treatments may be medical, such as IV injection of an antidote for drug overdose, or surgical such as inserting a chest tube for those with tension pneumothorax or hemothorax. While the above-mentioned steps are being carried out, it is crucial to continue chest compressions with minimal interruptions. This point is emphasized repeatedly in the new PALS guidelines because the key to successful PALS is proper BLS techniques.

In pediatric Assessment, the technique: EVALUATE-IDENTIFY-INTERVENE is usually employed. If the child is not breathing and there is no pulse, shout for help, start CPR, beginning with chest compressions. If a pulse is present, provide rescue breathing.

Assess		Action
Airway	Is the patient's airway open? Does the patient need an advanced airway?	Maintain an open airway via head tilt lift, OPA or NPA Advance airway maybe needed(LMA combitube or ET)
Breathing	Does the patient have adequate ventilation & oxygenation? Does the patient need an advanced airway? Is airway device properly placed and secure? Are exhaled CO2 & oxyhemoglobin saturation monitored?	Provide oxygen, assess adequacy. Determine if the placement of an advance airway outweighs the risk interrupting chest compressions. Confirm placement, security, and integrations of CPR & ventilation if advance airway is placed Continue to monitor exhaled CO2 levels
Circulation	What is the patient's initial and current cardiac rhythm? Is the access for drug & fluid administration established? Is the patient in need of fluid for resuscitation? Does the patient need drugs for rhythm or BP?	Establish IV/IO access. Attach ECG Administer drugs and IV/ IO fluids as appropriate
Differential Diagnosis	What was the underlying cause of cardiac arrest? Is the underlying cause reversible?	Identify and treat reversible causes

EKG interpretation and Pathology Recordings

Cardiac arrhythmias are due to the following mechanisms:

Arrhythmias of sinus origin - where electrical flow follows the usual conduction pathway but is too fast, too slow, or irregular. Normal sinus rate is 60-100 beats per minute. If the rate goes beyond 100 per minute, it is called sinus tachycardia. If the rate goes below 60 per minute, it is referred to as sinus bradycardia. *Ectopic rhythms* - electrical impulses originate from somewhere else other than the sinus node. *Conduction blocks* - electrical impulses go down the usual pathway but encounter blocks and delays.

Pre-excitation syndromes - the electrical impulses bypass the normal pathway and, instead, go down an accessory shortcut.

Randal (2004, p. 54) mentions that when interpreting electrocardiogram, it is important to identify the normal behavior of the heart, that is the baseline method. A heart in good condition will have a Normal Sinus Rhythm. Any deviation from a normal sinus rhythm is usually a thing of concern. Some deviations like sinus dysrhythmia are of low concern while rhythms like Ventricular fibrillation are life threatening emergencies. Let us take a look at some common EKG Strips.

Normal Sinus Rhythm

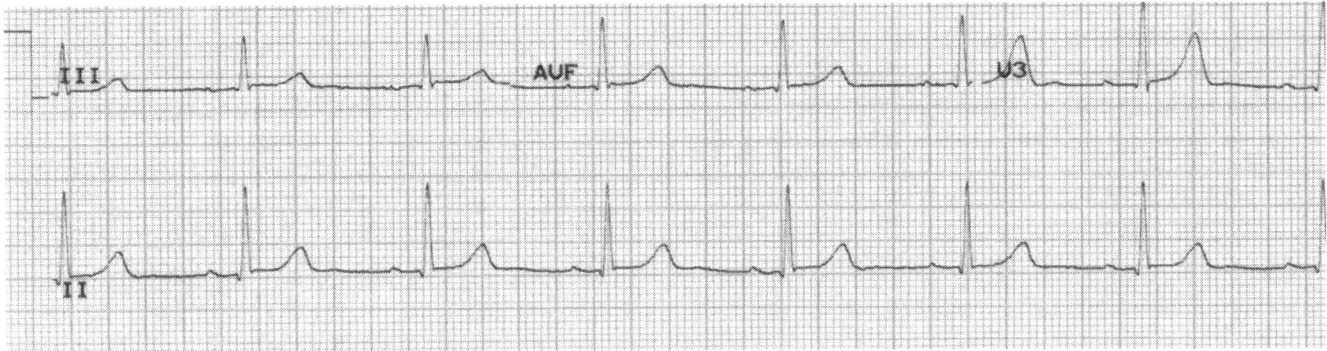

Originated from the SA Node and has the following characteristics:

a. Heart Rate of 60 – 100 bpm

b. Similar P waves in all the leads in front of all QRS complexes

c. A constant PR interval of 0.12 to 0.2 sec in all the leads,

d. Regular rhythm

e. QRS complex < 0.12

f. QT interval < 0.40

Sinus Bradycardia

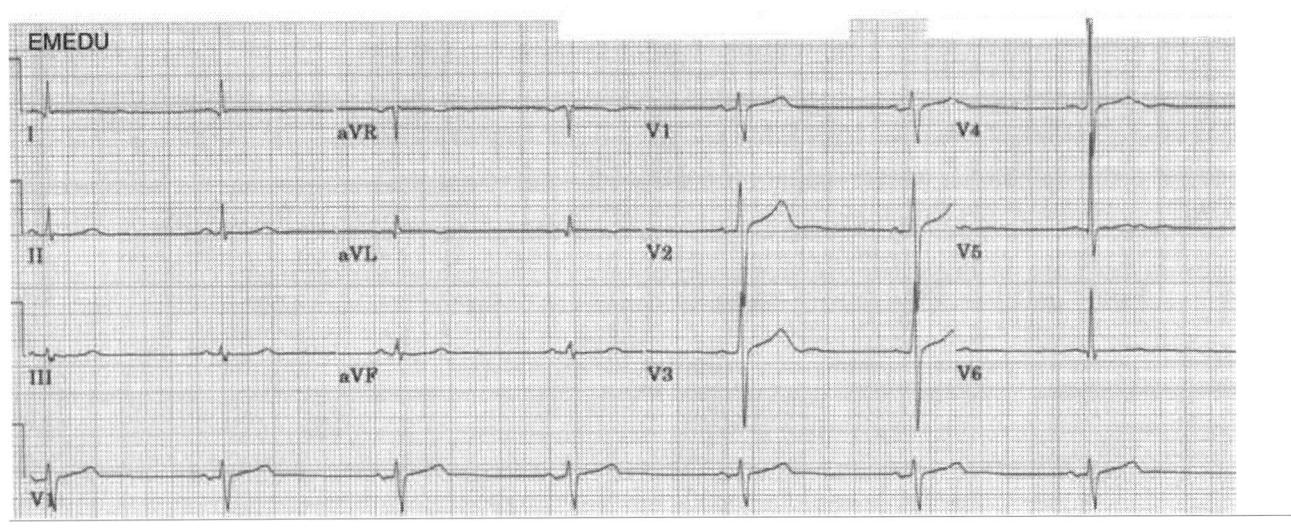

Bradycardia may be normal for athletes. It may also be normal in some individuals during sleep. Causes include vomiting, bearing down to have a bowel movement or diseases like myocardial infarction, obstructive jaundice and increased intracranial pressure. Medications such as digitalis, calcium-channel blockers and other anti-arrhythmic medications can also contribute to this rhythm. Features include:

a. HR less than 60 bpm

b. Normal equal P and QRS in all the leads, as well as normal PR intervals

c. . Bradycardia decreases the blood flow in the brain and other body tissues.

One can say that Sinus Bradycardia has the features of Normal Sinus Rhythm except a heart rate lower than 60 beats per minutes.

Sinus Tachycardia

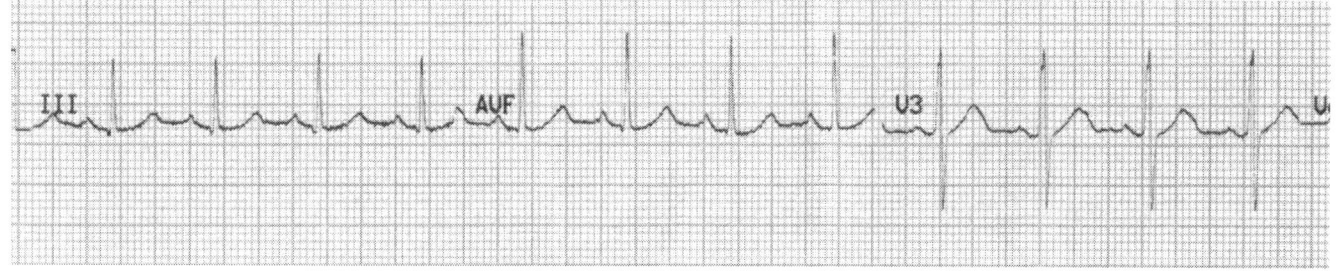

During stress and exercise, Sinus Tachycardia is normal. If Sinus Tachycardia persists at rest, conditions such as fever, dehydration, blood loss, anemia, anxiety, heart failure, hypermetabolic states and consumptions of stimulants such as cocaine, methamphetamine, etc. may be the cause. Drugs that can cause Sinus Tachycardia include: atropine, isoproterenol, epinephrine, dopamine, dobutamine, norepinephrine, nitroprusside and caffeine. Sinus Tach increases the heart's need for oxygen. Treatment includes finding out the underlying cause and treating it. Drugs of choice include: digitalis, beta-blockers, calcium-channel blockers, sedatives and other antiarrhythmic medications. Features include:

a. HR: 100 - 150 bpm

b. Normal equal P and QRS in all the leads, as well as normal PR intervals (0.12-0.20sec)

c. PR interval: 0.12-0.20 sec

d. QRS: < 0.12

Rhythm: Regular.

Sinus Tach originates from the SA Node.

Supraventricular Tachycardia (Life threatening)

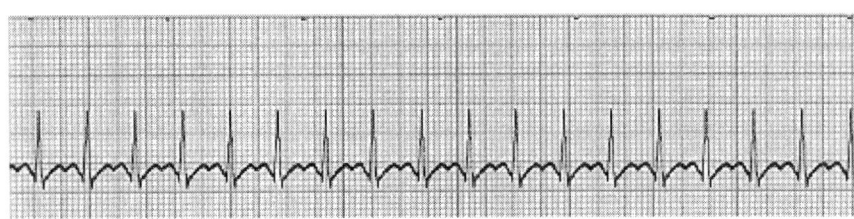

Atrial Tachycardia (AT) is caused by an irritable focus in the atria that fires electrical impulses after the normal firing of the SA node pacemaker. **HR is regular between 150 and 250 bpm.**

AV Reentry Tachycardia is caused when the electrical impulse passes through a passage other than AV node. Cardiac rhythm is regular but up to 250 bpm. P waves are often hidden by the QRS complexes or the QRS complexes that follow a P wave are different and with different PR interval (AV Nodal Reentry Tachycardia **AVNRT**).

In cases with **AV Reentry Tachycardia (AVRT) QRS** complexes are greater than 0.12 sec with a slurred up strike (delta wave) seen in one or more leads.

Atrial flutter

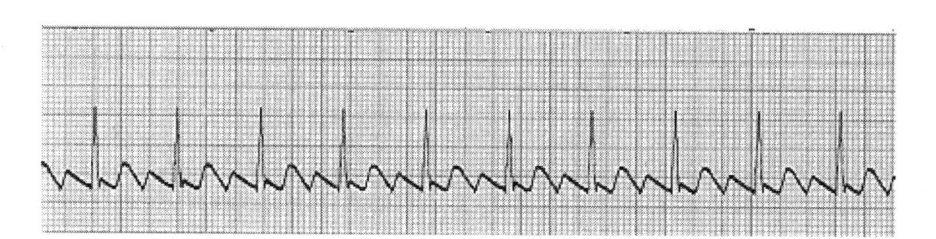

Atrial Flutter: Notice that there are no more "P" waves, instead a typical saw-tooth-like wave, called "F" wave is seen in the above recording. This rhythm leads to loss of atrial contraction resulting in decreased cardiac output 20-30%. Risks associated with this rhythm include: mural thrombi, hemodynamic instability, systemic or pulmonary embolism, etc. It is a life threatening situation. Cardioversion is usually done if it is an acute arrhythmia. If it is a chronic rhythm that is not responsive to medications, it is important that the patient be evaluated and possibly placed on an anticoagulant medication.

a. Atrial Flutter is characterized by rapid depolarization of a single atrial focus at a rate of 250-350 bpm.

b. Because the AV node cannot transmit every impulse at excessive rates, there is typically a slower ventricular rate (often appearing as a 2:1, 3:1, 4:1, etc. conduction ratio).

c. Typical **saw-toothed waves,** named "F" waves, followed by almost normal QRS complexes with a slower rate are seen in all the leads.

Atrial Fibrillation

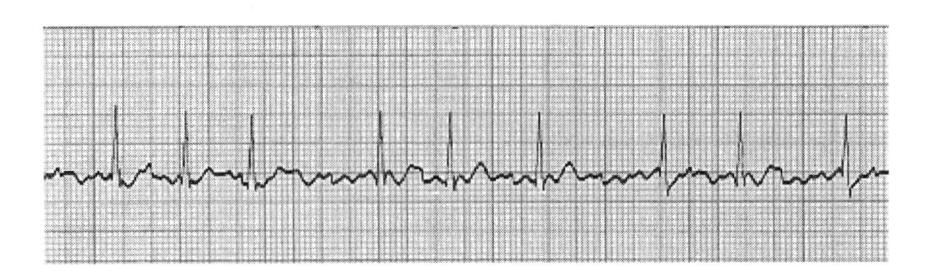

There are no "P" waves, instead they are substituted by small trembling waves, while QRST complex are almost normal and fired with a different rate.
Atrial fibrillation is caused by multiple irritable sites all over the atria firing at a rate exceeding 350 bpm. These rapid impulses cause quivering (fibrillation) of the muscular fibers, which results in a drastic decrease in the cardiac output, blood stagnation and the formation of a clot. Cardiac output is reduced with the loss of "Atrial Kick" because the atria are not contracting. If the ventricular rate are also fast, there will be further decreased cardiac output. The patient is at risk of pulmonary embolism or stroke. Causes: MI, Rheumatic Heart Disease, COPD, CHF, Ischemic Chest Trauma, CAD and open heart Surgery. Cardioversion is usually done in acute cases.

- No identifiable P waves can be seen, ***fibrillatory erratic "f" waves*** are seen in all the leads. Ventricular rhythm is very irregular, with a much slower rate than the atria. This is seen in all leads.

- Controlled atrial fibrillation: Average ventricular rate is less than 100 bpm.

- Uncontrolled atrial fibrillation: Average ventricular rate is over 100 bpm.

Premature Ventricular Complex

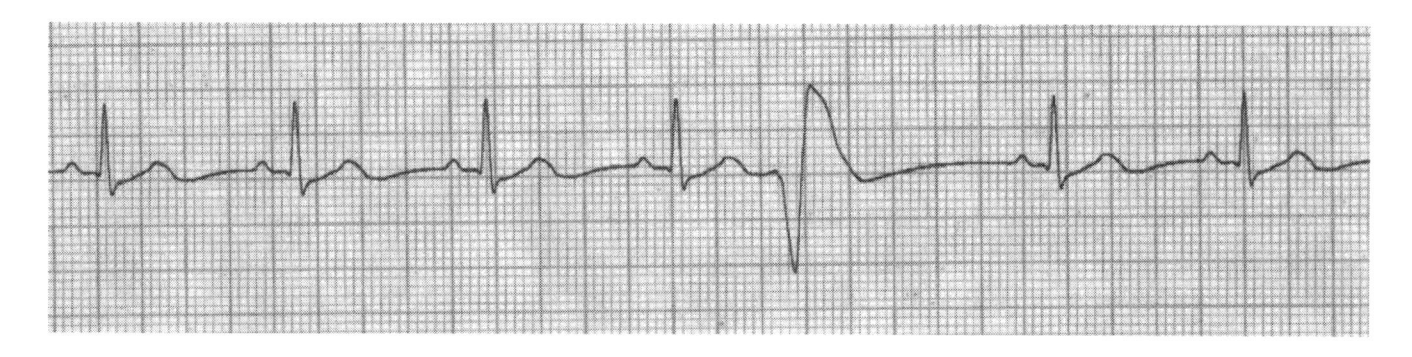

Notice the difference between the normal QRS complexes and the wide inverted abnormal QRS of the PVC and the full compensatory pause.

A premature ventricular complex arises from an irritable site within the ventricles. PVCs can appear as single, couplets, or triplets. Six or more PVCs occurring in a row are considered a run of V-Tach. PVC may appear in the same shape or in different shapes. When they appear in the same shape, they are believed to arise from a common point or focus, therefor are referred to as unifocal PVCs, but when they arise from different foci, they are referred to as multifocal PVCs.

The QRS of PVC is typically greater than 0.12 sec because the ventricular depolarization is abnormal or *aberrant*. The origin is usually ventricular/purkinje fibres. Causes: Increased catecholamines as seen in heightened emotions, stimulants such as coffee, nicotine, ethanol, cocaine, amphetamins, AMI, CHF, digitalis, increased vagal tones, hypoxia, acidosis, hypokalemia, hypomagnesemia, acidosis, ischemia, hypoxia and open heart surgery. T waves are usually in opposite direction of the QRS complex . A full compensatory pause usually follows a PVC. The rate and the PR interval are that of the underlying rhythm. The most important treatment is to find out and treat the underlying causes. Drugs of choice include beta blockers, procainamide, lidocaine, amiodarone, etc.

Ventricular Tachycardia

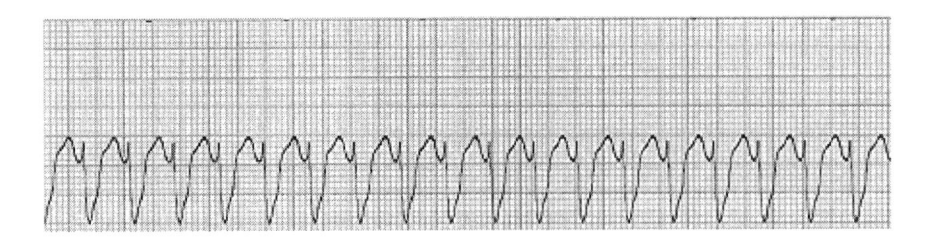

Ventricular Tachycardia (V-Tach) is characterized by 3 or more PVC's in a row at a rate over 100 bpm. If V-Tach occurs for more than 30 sec is called *sustained Ventricular Tachycardia*. The main characteristics of this rhythm are: Regular fast rhythm 100 to 250 bpm, No P waves or P waves may be present if SA node is functional, however, there is no relation to the QRS Wide, bizarre QRS complexes > 0.12 with T waves pointing in opposite direction from main QRS direction (T waves may be difficult to identify). If QRS complexes are different in size it is called *Polymorphic V-Tach* or "Torsades de Pointes".

Causes of V-Tach include hypoxia, acidosis, cardiomyopathy, mitral valve prolapse, digitalis toxicity, antiarrhythmics, electrolyte imbalance, liquid protein diets, increased intracranial pressure and central nervous system disorders. The longer a patient stays in V-Tach, the more difficult it is to convert to a normal rhythm. Stable patients may be medicated to attempt a chemical conversion. Unstable patients are treated promptly with defibrillation. **It is a life threatening emergency.**

Ventricular Fibrillation (Life threatening)

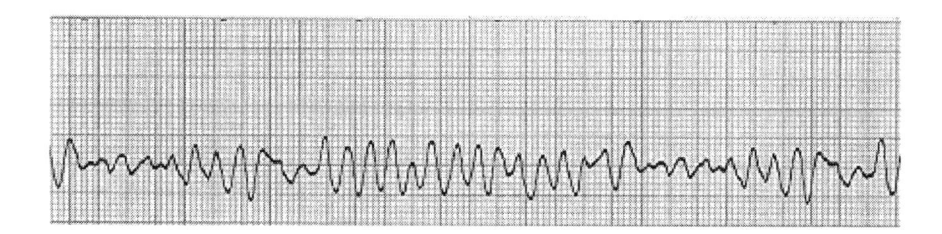

It is produced by multiple electrical sites firing electrical impulses at the same time resulting in quivering of the ventricles myocardial muscle fibers, but not a uniform contraction.

The rhythm is a chaotic deflection of different waves that vary in size, shape and duration. There are no normal visible waves. There is no contraction, there is no blood ejected in the blood vessels, so the blood can clot. This is a medical emergency, which requires defibrillation and CPR.

Asystole (No electrical activity in the heart)

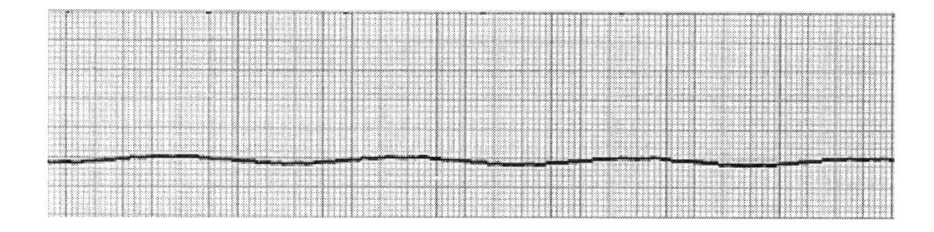

First Degree Heart Block, Type I

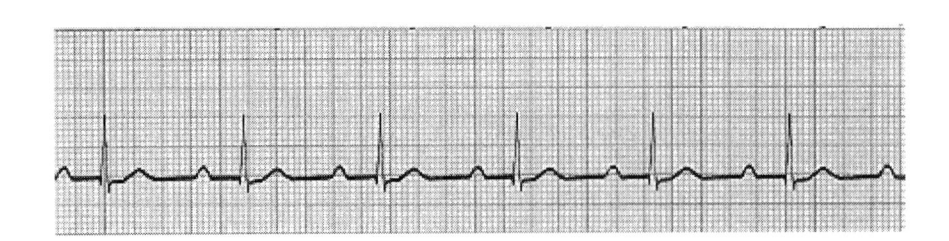

It is characterized by a delay of impulses at the level of AV node. . *PR interval is prolonged and is greater than 0.2 sec*

Second Degree Heart Block Type I

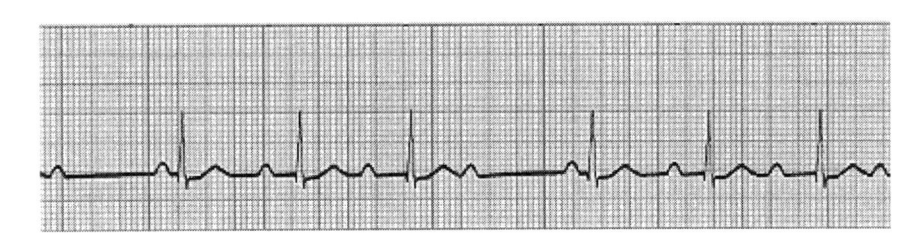

PR interval lengthens in each interval until one QRS disappears

Type II Second Degree AV Block (Mobitz II)
It is a more serious pathology.
Conducted P waves have a constant PR interval; but there are always non-conducted P waves between cardiac cycles, usually producing a "conduction ratio" between atria and ventricles (i.e. 2 P waves for each QRS, or 3 P waves for each QRS)

Third Degree AV Block. This type of AV block is also called a Complete Heart Block, or CHB, because impulses generated by the SA node are completely blocked before reaching the ventricular muscle fibers. The atria and ventricles beat independently from each other. Second degree blocks can progress in third degree blocks, especially after an inferior MI (myocardial Infarction). The third degree block's characteristics are:

-Atrial rate is greater than ventricular rate

-P waves are normal, there are no measurable PR intervals

-The atrial rhythm (P waves) is regular; AND the ventricular rhythm is regular (QRS complexes).

There is no relationship between P waves and QRS complexes

If the escape rhythm is junctional, the QRS complexes may appear normal in width and the ventricular rate may be slightly higher

If the escape rhythm is ventricular, the QRS complexes will be abnormally wide with a slower ventricular rate.

ACLS Scenario

The following section explains potentially life- threatening scenarios, stroke, respiration arrhythmias, and acute coronary syndrome, and their corresponding and recommended management techniques

1: Acute Stroke

There are two major types of stroke, *ischemic* and *hemorrhagic*. Ischemic stroke occurs 85% of all strokes cases and is a result of a blocked artery in the brain. Hemorrhagic stroke occur the remaining 15% of stroke cases and is the result of a ruptured blood vessel.

Recognizing stroke may be difficult because the signs of stroke are obscure and difficult. There is not a specific arrhythmia associated with stroke; however, an ECG may identify signs of atrial fibrillation, which could indicate the occurrence of a stroke. Other signs of stroke include confusion, difficulty seeing, walking, speaking or comprehending, severe headache, and numbness to one side of the body and lack of balance.

Stroke Assessment

7 Ds of Stroke

The steps to identify and treat stroke cases are referred to as the 7Ds of Stroke

> D1: Detection of stroke signs and symptoms
>
> D2: Dispatch EMS
>
> D3: Delivery of patient to a previously notified hospital that is prepared and able to deliver stroke care
>
> D4: Door of ED (Urgent triage in Emergency Department)
>
> D5: Data from CT scan

D6: Decision of the line of management

D7: Drug administration and monitoring

Out- of- Hospital Assessment Tools

AHA recommends that all emergency healthcare providers be trained in identifying the signs of stroke using the Cincinnati Pre-hospital Stroke Scale and the Los Angeles Pre-hospital Stroke Screen and tools

Cincinnati Prehospital Stroke Scale (CPSS) - This three part evaluation can be completed in a minute. Emergency personnel should have the patient perform all three tests and note the symptom. The more symptoms that the patient has, the greater the chance they are having a stroke. The table below outlines each test and possible outcomes.

Facial Droop (expose teeth or smile)	Arm Drift (close eyes, extended arms out palms up).	Abnormal Speech ("you can't teach old dog new tricks").
Normal- face moves the same on both sides	Normal- both arms move the same or not at all	Normal- speech is not slurred and correct

| Abnormal- movement is impaired on one side compared to the other | Abnormal- movement of one arm is impaired compared to the other. One arm may be lower than the other, even though the client tries to keep them at the same level. | Abnormal- speech is slurred, wrong or absent |

Los Angeles Pre-hospital Stroke Screen (LAPSS) - This evaluation uses test and patient's history in addition to the results of the CPSS evaluation, to identify patients with stroke. If patient meets all the criteria, then there is a 97% probability that they are having an acute stroke, and so needs to be immediately transported to a hospital. However, patients can have a stroke if not all criteria are met. The checklist below demonstrates 6 criteria, in which the possible outcomes are "yes" and "no". Treatment will be based on the results of the evaluation.

Criteria	Yes	Unknown	No
Age > 45 years old	x	x	x
No History of epileptic seizures	x	x	x

Symptom duration < 24 hours	x	x	x
Blood glucose between 60 and 400	x	x	x
Obvious Asymmetry (must be unilateral)	x	x	x
	Equal	Right Weak	Left Weak
Facial smile/ grimace	x	○ droop	○ Droop
Grip	x	○ Weak grip ○ No grip	○ Weak grip ○ No grip
Arm Strength	x	○ Drifts down ○ Falls rapidly	○ Drips down ○ Falls rapidly

The Stroke Chain of Survival

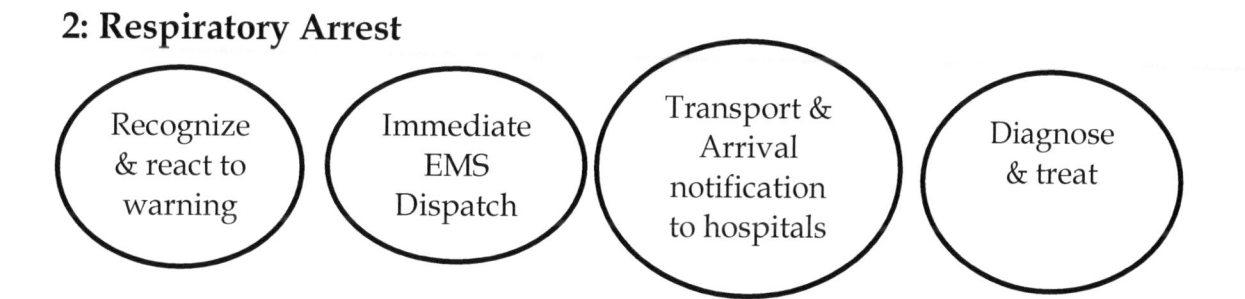

2: Respiratory Arrest

(Recognize & react to warning) (Immediate EMS Dispatch) (Transport & Arrival notification to hospitals) (Diagnose & treat)

In respiratory arrest situations, healthcare providers assess the scene, check patient response and activate EMS before beginning the ABCD's of BLS. The next steps are to open the patients airway and give 2 breaths if respirations are inadequate, look for carotid pulse (should take between 5 to 10 seconds) and attach defibrillator if patient does not have a pulse. The important factors to remember for respiratory cases are high- quality CPR, early defibrillation and reassessing the patient throughout the survey.

After primary survey has been completed, healthcare providers proceed to more advanced saving techniques, using the ACLS Secondary Survey as a guide. Healthcare providers are performing CPR, so any action that interrupts chest compressions need to be thoroughly evaluated before being implemented. If bag-mask ventilation is adequate, placing an advanced airway is postponed until the patient becomes unresponsive to initial resuscitation efforts. ACLS Survey Overview chart in this material can be used as a guide to providing resuscitation during the respiratory arrest.

Management Interventions

Both the BLS and ACLS interventions are used in managing respiratory arrest. The basic ABCs are assessed and completed, in addition to providing suctioning and ventilation with advance airways, Healthcare providers should avoid hyperventilation when providing assisted ventilation. Hyperventilation increases airway pressure and PEEP (Positive End Expiratory Pressure), which can then lead to an increased cerebral venous and intracranial pressures. This string of events leads to an overall increase in brain ischemia.

Part of the ABCs is to maintain oxygen saturation ≥90% and airway patency. To maintain patency, the head tilt-chin lift maneuver can be implemented, or if patient is suspected with cervical trauma the jaw thrust without head extension maneuver should be used. To help maintain airway the healthcare providers can insert an oropharyngeal or nasopharyngeal airway. The chart compares the difference between OPA and NPA device.

OPA vs. NPA

	Oropharyngeal Airway (OPA)	Nasopharyngeal Airway (NPA)
Device & Placement	J- Shaped; Placed over the tongue	Rubber or plastic uncuffed Through nostril, along the nasal floor
Applications	• Unconscious patients • When head tilt & jaw thrust are in effective • To keep airway open during bag-mask ventilation • During suctioning in intubated patients	• Conscious and semiconscious • Intact gag & cough reflex • When OPA insertion is hard or not possible • Neurologically impaired patient w/ upper airway obstruction
Insertion	• Clear mouth & pharynx	• Choose correct device

Technique	• Choose correct device size • Insert device • Rotate device 180° as it approaches the pharynx posterior wall	size • Lubricate airway • Insert device
Precautions	• Incorrect size can cause trauma or obstruct airway • Insert smoothly to avoid tissue damage	• Incorrect size can cause gastritis • Insert smoothly to avoid tissue • Device may cause vomiting • Improper placement

The suctioning management technique is used for patients in respiratory arrest, and the airway patency. Suctioning should be performed to remove blood, vomit or excessive secretions within the airway. There are two types of suctioning catheters available, soft and rigid. Soft are used to suction the patient's nose or mouth and ET tube deep suctioning. Rigid catheters are used to clear out the patient's oropharynx, especially for thicker substances.

Advanced airway ventilation typically leverages a combitube, LMA or ET tubes (Laryngeal Mask Airway and Endotracheal). The correct device is dependent upon the skills of the resuscitation team and the resources available. Only experienced healthcare providers should attempt advanced airway placement. Combitubes are alternative to ET tubes and provide adequate ventilation. LMA devices are difficult to insert; therefore, bag-mask ventilation can be used as an alternative. LMA are also an alternative to ET tubes and provide similar ventilation support. Once an advance airway is in place, CPR protocol changes. Healthcare providers are now advised to deliver one breath every 5 seconds (about 8-10 breaths/ minute) and no longer required to interrupt chest compressions for ventilations.

Ventilation Protocol

-Ventilate once every 5-6 seconds (10-12/ minute)

-Each breath over 1 second

-Make the chest rise with each breath given.

Acute Coronary Syndromes

Acute coronary Syndromes (ACS) is a term used to categorize a spectrum of diseases that affects the heart, such as acute myocardial infarction (AMI) and unstable angina (UA)

Pathophysiology

ACS develops through several symptoms, and it starts with the build-up of unstable plaque. Plaque is the most common cause of ACS. When excessive amounts of plaque builds up, it can rupture thus, activating the coagulation system with thrombin generation. If thrombus is partially occluded, it produces symptoms of ischemia and if it is periodically occluded it can cause myocardial necrosis leading to NSTEMI (Non-ST segment elevation Myocardial Infarction. Progression to a larger clot that completely blocks the thrombus will eventually result in STEMI (ST-segment elevation myocardial infarction).

Management Interventions

The goals of ACS therapy are to quickly identify patients with STEMI, perform rapid resuscitation therapy, relieve ischemic pain, prevent major adverse cardiac events (MACE) and treat life-threatening complications (unstable tachycardia, symptomatic bradycardia, VF/ pulseless VT). Successful and effective interventions need to occur within the first hour that the symptoms began.

Management begins with recognizing patient's chest discomfort, which can suggest ischemia. Healthcare providers should be looking for discomfort in the chest, which can progress to the shoulders and back, pressure or fullness causing discomfort, and sudden shortness of breaths are signs of ACS. Hopefully, EMS will be dispatched as quickly as possible. If they are authorized, they should recommend that the patient chew on aspirin (if not allergic or doesn't have GI bleeding) as EMS team arrives.

ACS Drug Treatment

- Use of oxygen, aspirin, nitroglycerin and morphine are recommended for patients who present with ischemic chest pain
- Contraindications of aspirin → allergy, recent GI bleed
- Contraindications of nitroglycerin and morphine →hypotension

STEMI Therapy

Reperfusion therapy provided within the first hour of symptoms reduces the risk of mortality. Reperfusion therapy is the preferred treatment for STEMI patients, especially within the first 12 hours of onset of symptoms. Fibrinolytic therapy and PCI are two types of reperfusion therapy; fibrinolytics is the preferred treatment and PCI (Percutaneous Coronary Intervention) is an alternative. Patient's clinical condition must fit the outlined in the fibrinolytic checklist before therapy can be performed.

In fibrinolytic therapy, a clot- busting, fibrinoltic agent is administered to patients present with STEMI symptoms without contraindications. It is not recommended for patients after the 12-hour mark, but can be administered if patient is still presenting ischemic chest pain. It is not recommended for patients with ST- segments depression or after 24 hours from onset of symptoms unless posterior MI is a possibility. Door- to- needle time of less than 30 minutes is preferred. An alternative to fibrinoltic therapy, PCI is used when patients are unresponsive to fibrinolytic therapy. Coronary angioplasty is the most important form of PCI. PCI is preferred when patient has contraindications to fibrinolytic therapy and most effective if preferred between 3-12 hours from symptoms onset. Door- to- balloon time of less than 90 minutes is preferred.

Adjunct treatments such as IV nitroglycerin and heparin are also useful in STEMI patients.

The chart below outlines the applicable uses of each drug.

	Indications	**Management**
IV Nitroglycerin	1. Chest discomfort (not responsive to SL, nitroglycerin spray or morphine) 2. Pulmonary edema & hypertension causing complications in STEMI	1. Titrate to effect, SBP> 90mm or no less than 300mm HG below 2. Titrate to effect, SBP no less than 30mm hg below baseline (hypotension) & no less than 10mm hg(normotensive)
Heparin	1. Administered during PCI & fiberinolytic therapies 2. LV mural thrombus 3. Atrial fibrillation	1. Doses are dependent on specific strategies

Common Cardiovascular Agents

One of the essentials of quality care of a patient who is having an acute myocardial infarction is pharmacological therapy. The following are the common pharmacological agents used.

Oxygen

Oxygen should be given to all patients with acute chest pain that may be due to cardiac ischemia, suspected hypoxemia of any cause, and cardiopulmonary arrest. Prompt treatment of the hypoxemia may prevent cardiac arrest. For patients breathing spontaneously, masks and nasal cannulas can be used to administer oxygen.

Epinephrine

Epinephrine is indicated in the management of cardiac arrest. The chance of successful defibrillation is enhanced by administration of epinephrine and proper oxygenation.

Isoproterenol (Isuprel)

Isoproterenol produces an overall increase in heart rate and myocardial contractility, but newer agents have replaced it in most clinical settings. It is contraindicated in the routine treatment of cardiac arrest.

Dopamine (Intropin)

Dopamine is indicated for significant hypotension in the absence of hypovolemia. Significant hypotension is present when systolic blood pressure is less than 90 mmHg with evidence of poor tissue perfusion, oliguria, or changes in mental status. It should be used at the lowest dose that produces adequate perfusion of vital organs.

Beta Blockers: Propranolol, Metoprolol, Atenolol, and Esmolol

Beta blockers reduce heart rate, blood pressure, myocardial contractility, and myocardial oxygen consumption which make them effective in the treatment of angina pectoris and hypertension.

They are also useful in preventing atrial fibrillation, atrial flutter, and paroxysmal supraventricular tachycardia. Adverse effects of beta blockers are hypotension, congestive heart failure and broncho-spasm.

Lidocaine

Lidocaine is the drug of choice for the suppression of ventricular ectopy, including ventricular tachycardia and ventricular flutter. Excessive doses can produce neurological changes, myocardial depression, and circulatory depression. Neurological toxicity is manifested as drowsiness, disorientation, decreased hearing ability, paresthesia, and muscle twitching, and

eventual seizures.

Verapamil

Verapamil is used in the treatment of paroxysmal supraventricular tachycardia (PSVT), effective in terminating more than 90% of episodes of PVST in adults and infants. Verapamil is also useful in slowing ventricular response to atrial flutter and fibrillation. Vigilant monitoring of blood pressure is recommended due to hypotension that could occur.

Digitalis

Digitalis increases the force of cardiac contraction as well as cardiac output.. Digitalis toxicity is common with an incidence of up to 20%. Patients require constant monitoring for signs and symptoms of toxicity such as: yellow vision, nausea, vomiting, and drowsiness.

Morphine Sulfate

It is the traditional drug of choice for the pain and anxiety associated with acute myocardial infarction. In high doses, morphine sulfate may cause respiratory depression. It is a controlled substance and has a tendency for abuse and addiction.

Nitroglycerin

Nitroglycerin is a powerful smooth muscle relaxant effective in relieving angina pectoris. It is effective for both exertional and rest angina. Headache is a common consequence following the administration of this drug. Hypotension may occur and patients should be instructed to sit or lie down while taking nitroglycerin.

More Information on Stroke and Myocardial infarction

Stroke

Causes

The human brain is the center and origin of all processes taking place in the body. For this reason, the head should be handled with care so that no damage occurs and affects operations in the brain. However some circumstances may be unavoidable making humans susceptible to situations that are injurious. Stroke is a kind of disease that affects the human brain and when not attended to on time, it can lead to total loss of life. This condition is sometimes referred to as cerebrovascular disease (CVA) or cerebral hemorrhage.

There are two commonly known types of stroke that human beings can be affected by; Ischemic stroke is a kind of brain attack that arises when a vessel which transports blood to human brain is blocked by the blood clotting process (Richard, et al, 2009). In this case, the clot creates a barricade, blocking the routine flow of blood. This occurs in two main ways; first there can be a blood clot happening in a brain artery which happens to be very narrow, this process is referred to as *"Thrombotic stroke."* Secondly, there may be a case where a clot breaks off from a completely different location.

Alternatively, the blood clot can be transported to the blood vessels in the brain from a different part of the body, in both cases; the clot is a barrier blood flow in the brain. In the condition, the kind of stroke suffered from is referred to as *"embolism"* or *"embolic stroke"*

Another kind of stroke happens when a weak blood vessel happens to burst in the brain. This makes the blood to start leaking into the brain against the normal way that the brain is intended to function (Kenning, et al, 2012). In both cases, death is always knocking for the victim in the case urgent effective medical care is not administered.

Pathophysiology

When a person is affected by stroke, the kind of symptoms that are exhibited depends on the part of the brain that have been affected. It is possible for someone to experience the symptoms without being able to know that its stroke. People should be aware that symptoms of stroke develop unexpectedly and without due warning. For the first few days the symptoms occur on and off, making it hard for one to explain the prevailing body condition. When stroke first occurs, its symptoms are said to be very severe, however, this effects gets worse as time continues.

If bleeding happens in the brain, the victim experiences headaches which start as mild but soon become severe. These headaches are prevalent when the victim is lying flat; the severity of the headaches wakes up the victim from sleep. The victim feels severe headaches especially when he changes his position when sleeping, when he happens to bend or if he coughs.

The severity of the brain attack and its specific position determine the kind of symptoms experienced. However, most of them include; general modification in general attentiveness, changes in hearing and taste habits of the victim. At the same time, the victim may experience changes which may affect his ability to touch or feel pain; however, the victim needs to seek urgent medical diagnosis in order to ascertain the real cause of symptoms, as having these symptoms may not necessary mean that an individual is suffering from stroke.

Management

Stroke is always a serious medical case which requires urgent medical attention; otherwise it is a potential cause of death to the victims who suffer from it (Brown, 2001). Only a trained medical practitioner is in a better position to handle brain attack using various types of interventions or surgery in critical cases. When the stroke being experienced is a result of a blood clot, the medical practitioner can offer a drug which bursts up the clot (anticoagulant) and normal blood flow resumes. This treatment needs to be induced within 3-4 hours after experiencing the initial symptoms. Other ways of effective managment are determined by the specific causes of stroke.

When the patient is taken to hospital, doctors will decide on the kind of therapy that the victim will be put to. That is the 6th D of stroke intervention. If the stroke progresses, depending on symptoms, the victim could be put on occupational therapy, speech or physical, all of which have to be approved by a qualified medical doctor.

Myocardial infarction

Causes

One of the most dangerous conditions that leads to termination of human life is heart attack. The heart is an essential body organ with the function of upholding the life of each and every living organism. As an important organ, it has one main function; to pump blood. When the heart stops functioning, the body lacks the much needed oxygen, something that suffocates body cells leading to death of the victim. Myocardial infarction is a condition where the human heart lacks oxygen as a result of blockage of normal blood flow to the myocardial muscles. This deadly condition is also referred to as heart attack in common terms.

The heart is supplied with oxygenated blood from two main vessels referred to as coronary arteries. When either of the arteries is blocked for any particular reason; the heart suffers from lack of oxygen. This condition of attack to the heart is known as *"Cardiac ischemia,"* which is dangerous since when it happens without prior warning, it causes suffocation of heart muscle cells, leading to the death of the portion of the myocardium it occurs. The death of tissues is called tissue necrosis or tissue 'infarction'. Since in this case it occurs in the myocardial cells, it is called myocardial infarction or popularly (MI).

Pathophysiology

Heart attack has been cited as one of the most dangerous conditions, this means that individuals should always seek medical attention as soon as they are able to identify any symptoms that could be associated with the attack (Heart Disease Health Center, 2014). Symptoms of heart attack are sometimes rare or difficult to ascertain. This means that any abnormal body experiences should be diagnosed medically with due urgency. In general, heart attack symptoms are often associated with pains in the chest which run from mild to severe.

Some victims experience difficulties in breathing accompanied by experiences of dizziness, fainting or sometimes nausea. At the initial stages, a victim of heart attack can easily mistake it for heart burn. Usually the pains in the heart appear to be constant in some cases while it is intermittent at other times. Medical research has shown that women have fewer chances of getting heart attacks compared to men.

On average, there are close to 25% of cases of heart attacks which occur without showing any possible signs. These kinds of attacks are usually associated with *"silent ischemia"* a condition that is characterized by infrequent interruptions of the normal flow of blood into the heart. Something peculiar about these attacks is that they are associated with less or no pains, however, their effect is the same, they are lethal and can result in the death of the victim.

Management

Most of the victims of heart attacks die before they get the much needed medical attention in hospitals and other reliable medical practitioners. Early treatment mechanisms are aimed at reducing severity of damage to the victim's heart. This is only possible if action is taken in due time to save the victim. When a person suspects that he is having a heart attack, there are medicines which can be administered immediately to reduce potential harm. Some of the medicines include aspirin which is helpful in thinning blood (NIH, n.d), hence reducing its ability to clot. Other common interventions include treating of chest pains and use of nitroglycerin medicine in order to decrease the hearts workload and enhance normal flow of blood in the coronary arteries.

After medical diagnosis has been established by doctors, immediate treatment is begun so as to bring back normal blood flow to the heart muscles. Two main strategies are used in the management of heart attack. One of the methods is using medicine aimed at bursting possible blood clots in the arteries (Anticoagulants). Anticoagulants are very effective; however, they ought to be used with 3-4 hours from detecting the first symptoms. Another effective method to treat heart attack is the use of PCI (Percutaneous Coronary Intervention). This method does not require any surgical processes but effectively opens arteries that are blocked are have become narrow, reducing normal blood flow to the heart.

In administering this treatment mechanism, a thin flexible tube that has a balloon on one end or a related device is inserted into a blood vessel in the groin area up to the narrowed artery or one that is blocked. After it has been inserted in the blood vessel, the balloon or other device are filled with air so that they are compressed on the wall of the blood vessel. This process resumes normal flow of blood in the arteries, something that reduces the effect of heart attack. People should always pay attention to any symptoms in their bodies since they may be potential causes of death when not attended to urgently.

Once again, thanks for purchasing this book. You may also like my BLS for Healthcare Professionals Student Manual

http://www.amazon.com/dp/B00J2GKSKU.

References

Brown, M. B. (2001). Identification and Management of Difficult Stroke and Tia Syndromes. *Journal of Neurology, Neurosurgery Psychiatry.* 70(1):**17-22**

Heart Disease Health Center (2014). *Understanding Heart Attack: The Basics.* Retrieved from, < http://www.webmd.com/heart-disease/understanding-heart-attack-basics>

Kenning, et al, (2012). Cranial decompression for the treatment of malignant intracranial hypertension after ischemic cerebral infarction: decompressive craniectomy and hinge craniotomy. *Journal of neurosurgery.* 116(6):1289-98.

NIH, (n.d). *How Is a Heart Attack Treated?* Retrieved from, < http://www.nhlbi.nih.gov/health/health-topics/topics/heartattack/treatment.html>

Richard, E. L, et al (2009). Recommendations for imaging of acute ischemic stroke: a scientific statement from the American Heart Association. STROKE. 40:346-367.

PALS Manual Review Questions

Section One

1) What are the keys to a successful code team?
    a. Teamwork, submission, punctuality
    b. Communication, teamwork, respect
    c. Respect, punctuality, knowledge
    d. None of the above

2) When a team works together it:
    a. Increases pay rates
    b. Increases customer satisfaction
    c. Increases the chance of successful resuscitation
    d. Increases number of return customers

3) Who should take the commanding role in the resuscitation team?
    a. Team leader
    b. A family member
    c. The home health agent
    d. Someone in the hallway

4) Who is best qualified to be a team leader?
    a. Someone who is good at chest compressions
    b. Someone who is comfortable with AEDs
    c. Someone who has read all of the books
    d. Someone who is experienced in all areas of resuscitation

5) How should messages be communicated amongst the team?
    a. Shouting loudly
    b. Calmly, concisely, and in a straightforward manner
    c. In whispers so as not upset the patient
    d. In writing

6) If you do not understand something you should:
    a. Smile and nod
    b. Pretend that you heard it and make something up
    c. Nothing

    d. Ask the person to repeat what he/she said

7) When assigning tasks:
    a. Assign all of them to the best team member
    b. Let people volunteer
    c. Assign tasks evenly and appropriately
    d. None of the above

8) You are asked to perform a task that you have never done before. You should:
    a. Speak up and notify the team leader that the task is above your skillset
    b. Attempt to perform the task
    c. Tell the person next to you to do the task
    d. Walk out of the room

9) When does assessment of the patient need to happen?
    a. Before resuscitation efforts
    b. Throughout resuscitation efforts
    c. After resuscitation efforts
    d. Assessment is optional

10) What does BLS stress?
    a. Later Rescue breaths and Later defibrillation
    b. Early Rescue breaths and Later compressions
    c. Later compressions and Later rescue breaths
    d. Early CPR and early defibrillation

11) Which of the following is a goal of BLS?
    a. Restoring oxygen ventilation
    b. Maintaining artificial circulation
    c. Sustaining the patient until ACLS or PALS can be started
    d. All of the above

12) Before starting BLS or PALS, you should:
    a. Make sure that the scene is safe
    b. Begin chest compressions
    c. Defibrillate
    d. Start oxygen

13) How many steps make up BLS?
   a. 6
   b. 4
   c. 3
   d. 2

14) To remember the steps you should remember:
   a. ABCDE
   b. CABE
   c. CABD
   d. BEADC

15) When checking for responsiveness you should:
   a. Tap and shout
   b. Watch for chest movement
   c. Check for breathing
   d. All of the above

16) The second step is to:
   a. Check the carotid pulse
   b. Activate the emergency response system
   c. Start rescue breaths
   d. Start chest compressions

17) The third step is circulation. Which of the following is not involved handling the circulation phase?
   a. Check pulse on the carotid
   b. Begin chest compressions
   c. Tap and shout
   d. Switch providers every two minutes

18) If you do not find a pulse within ___ seconds start compressions.
   a. 20 seconds
   b. 10 seconds
   c. 15 seconds
   d. 30 seconds

19) PALS begins with:
   a. Analyzing circulation with a manual defibrillator

b. Compressions
   c. IV fluids and medications
   d. All of the above

20) PALS also includes:
   a. IV fluids and medications
   b. Placement of airway devices
   c. Continuing chest compressions
   d. All of the above

21) Your task is almost finished and you notice that your coworker needs help. You should:
   a. Attempt to finish your task while you help your coworker
   b. Shout at the person not doing anything
   c. Calmly and clearly point out that your coworker needs help
   d. Let the coworker deal with it

22) What should your primary focus be?
   a. Your task
   b. Consoling family members
   c. Performing your job as fast as possible
   d. Providing quality patient care

23) A patient needs resuscitation. Several of the people in the room are new and have questions. You should:
   a. Patiently repeat yourself when they ask
   b. Speak over them
   c. Tell them to figure out the answer themselves
   d. Ignore the newbies

24) Everyone is part of the resuscitation team. This means that:
   a. You should be only concerned with your professional advancement
   b. There will never be conflict
   c. Each member is expected to perform on his/her own
   d. Every part of the team is expected to help the other

25) You do not agree with a course of action that your team member took in the last resuscitation attempt. The resuscitation attempt is now over. You should:

a. Share your thoughts and ideas in a constructive, non-confrontational manner
b. Avoid being on that person's team next time
c. Nothing
d. Confrontationally tell the other member she/he was wrong

26) During a resuscitation someone should:
a. Keep a log of the medications and reactions to them
b. Keep a log of the resuscitation efforts
c. Continually review the resuscitation load
d. All of the above

27) What does BLS stress?
a. Later Rescue breaths and Later defibrillation
b. Early Rescue breaths and Later compressions
c. Later compressions and Later rescue breaths
d. Early CPR and early defibrillation

28) Which of the following is a systematic approach to basic life support that any trained healthcare provider performs?
a. BLS
b. CABD
c. ACLS
d. ABCD

29) Which of the following is the main difference between PALS and BLS?
a. PALS excludes chest compressions focusing only on rescue breaths
b. PALS allows the team leader to decide when to defibrillate based on reading heart rhythms
c. BLS allows the team leader to decide when to defibrillate based on heart rhythms
d. BLS begins by defibrillating as the first step

30) Basic resuscitation efforts have failed. Your team then:
a. Determine that the patient is dead
b. Call a doctor
c. Continue with PALS
d. None of the above

31) Another difference between PALS and BLS is that:
a. Medication can be given during PALS in order to improve chances of resuscitation
b. Open heart massaging is an option
c. BLS is for common people while PALS is for anyone in a healthcare setting
d. None of the above

32) You are attempting to resuscitate a patient. The patient has a pneumothorax and requires a chest tube. What kind of resuscitation efforts would help this patient?
a. BLS
b. PALS
c. DLS
d. EMLS

33) When determining whether or not to use and advanced airway you should:
a. Determine whether or not the patient would want an advanced airway
b. Check the patient's chart
c. Determine if the placement of the airway outweighs the risk of stopping compressions
d. Call a respiratory therapist

34) During the differential diagnosis:
a. Perform compressions
b. Determine how long before the patient recovers
c. Determine what could have been done differently by the team
d. Determine what caused the cardiac arrest and treat reversible causes

35) In order to open an airway during BLS you should:
a. Use head tilt and chin lift
b. Intubate
c. Use an advanced airway
d. All of the above

36) Where is the proper place to check the pulse?
a. The jugular vein
b. The carotid
c. The supraventricular artery

d. The inside of the thigh

37) Following defibrillation you should:
a. Immediately start rescue breaths
b. Immediately resume compressions
c. Immediately shock again
d. Immediately provide an advanced airway

38) PALS often begins with:
a. Analyzing the heart rhythms
b. Reading the chart
c. Checking for the carotid pulse
d. Calling the doctor

39) If the patient is not breathing you should:
a. Provide immediate shock
b. Check the airway
c. Begin compressions
d. Intubate

40) After ten seconds you have not found a pulse. You should:
a. Defibrillate
b. Perform a rescue breath
c. Begin compressions
d. Transport the patient to the ER

Section Two

41) What is a normal sinus rate?
a. 20-60 bpm
b. 60-100 bpm
c. 100-120 bpm
d. 120-140 bpm

42) What is an arrhythmia of sinus origin?
   a. When electrical flow is disrupted and originates in the ventricles
   b. When the electrical flow is disrupted, but is still a normal heart rate
   c. When the electrical flow is stopped
   d. When the electrical flow is normal, but the heart rate is too fast or slow

43) What is an ectopic rhythm?
   a. When the electrical flow is normal, but the beat is irregular
   b. When the electrical flow is normal, but the heartbeat is too fast
   c. When the electrical flow originates from anywhere other than the sinus node
   d. None of the above

44) A heart rate with a normal electrical flow, but more than 100 BPM is called:
   a. Sinus tachycardia
   b. Ventricular fibrillation
   c. Sinus bradycardia
   d. Ventricular tachycardia

45) A heart rate with normal electrical flow, but fewer than 60 bpm is called:
   a. Sinus tachycardia
   b. Ventricular fibrillation
   c. Sinus bradycardia
   d. Ventricular tachycardia

46) What is a conduction block?
   a. The foundation for electrical impulse
   b. A type of brick used to build cardiac wards
   c. Blocks or delays along electrical pathways
   d. All of the above

47) What is a pre-excitation syndrome?
   a. Electrical impulses bypassing normal electrical pathways
   b. A type of sinus rhythm
   c. A block or delay among electrical pathways
   d. A type of tachycardia

48) The following is an example of

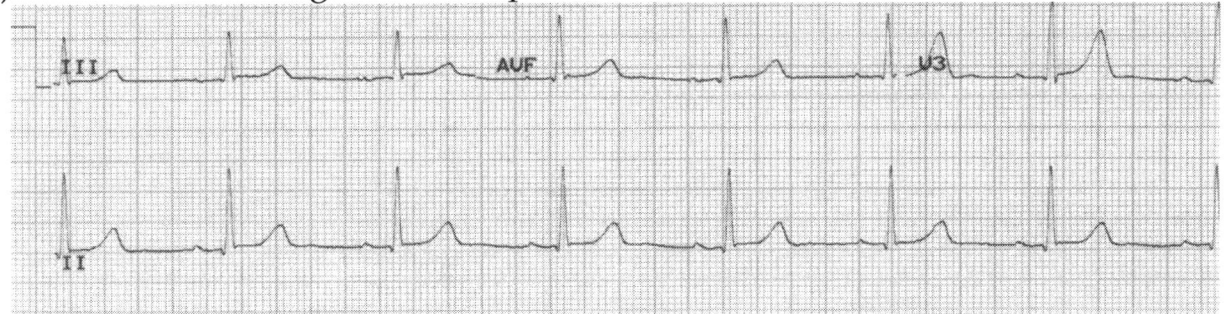

a. Pre-excitation syndrome
b. A block or delay
c. A normal sinus rhythm
d. Atrial fibrillation

49) Which of the following is not a part of a normal sinus rhythm?
a. 60-100 BPM
b. QRS complex < 0.12
c. Regular rhythm
d. Unique P waves in the front of all QRS complexes

50) Which of the following statements about bradycardia is false?
a. It is a heart rate of less than 60 BPM
b. It is characterized by normal equal P and QRS in all leads
c. It shows the characteristics of normal sinus rhythms
d. It is never normal in any person

51) When is sinus tachycardia normal?
a. When a person becomes elderly
b. Never
c. During stress and exercise
d. During rest

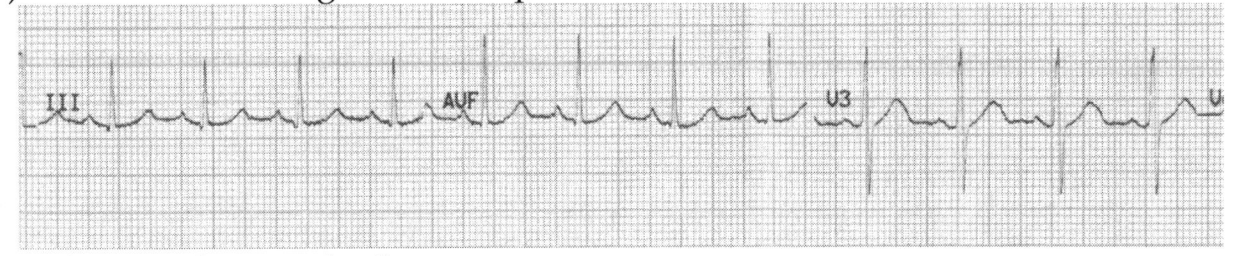

52) The following is an example of

a. A normal sinus rhythm
b. Sinus tachycardia

c. Sinus Bradycardia
   d. Supraventricular Tachycardia

53) The following is an example of

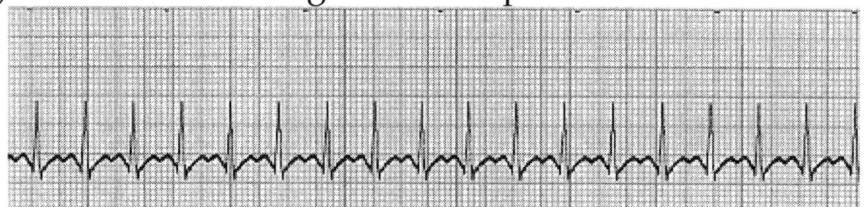

   a. A normal sinus rhythm
   b. Sinus tachycardia
   c. Sinus bradycardia
   d. Supraventricular Tachycardia

54) A saw-tooth like wave called "F" wave that causes a 20%-30% decrease in cardiac output is called:
   a. Supraventricular Tachycardia
   b. AV reentry Tachycardia
   c. Atrial flutter
   d. Atrial fibrillation

55) Atrial fibrillation is characterized by:
   a. Small trembling waves rather than "P" waves
   b. Defined "P" waves, but no "S" waves
   c. Small trembling waves rather than "T" waves
   d. None of the above

56) Which of the following is characterized by 3 or more PVC's in a row?
   a. Atrial tachycardia
   b. Ventricular tachycardia
   c. Asystole
   d. Premature ventricular complex

57) Which of the following is produced because of multiple electrical sites firing at the same time, causing quivering?
   a. Asystole
   b. Ventricular fibrillation
   c. Atrial fibrillation

d. Ventricular tachycardia

58) When the PR interval is longer than 0.2 seconds it is:
a. First degree heart block, type I
b. Third degree heart block, type I
c. Second degree heart block, type III
d. Fourth degree heart block, type II

59) A complete heart block is also known as:
a. A second degree AV block
b. A third degree aneurism
c. A first degree ventricular block
d. A third degree AV block

60) Which of the following shows an inverted QRS with a full compensatory pause?
a. A second degree AV block
b. Asystole
c. A premature ventricular complex
d. Sinus bradycardia

61) A normal sinus rhythm should have a QRS complex that is:
a. Less than 0.5
b. Less than 0.10
c. Less than 0.12
d. Greater than 0.12

62) The following is an example of

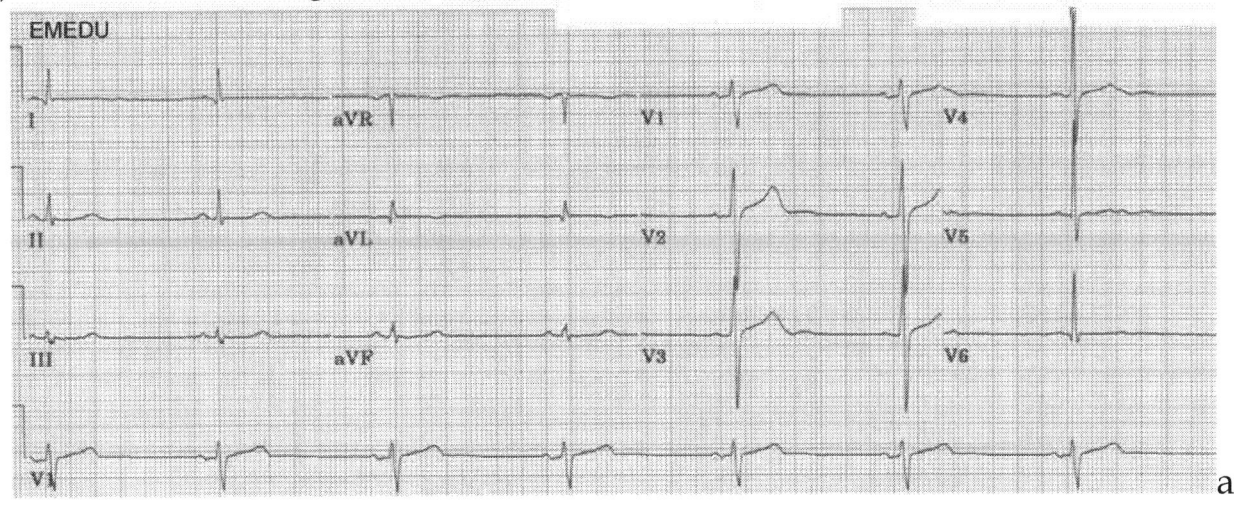

a. Sinus tachycardia
b. Sinus bradycardia
c. Ventricular tachycardia
d. Ventricular bradycardia

63) Which of the following causes sinus bradycardia?
a. Obstructive jaundice
b. Vomiting
c. Increased intracranial pressure
d. All of the above

64) Which of the following causes sinus tachycardia?
a. Exercise
b. Caffeine
c. Heart failure
d. All of the above

65) Which of the following statements about supraventricular tachycardia is false?
a. The heart rate is between 150 and 250 BPM
b. It is caused by an irritable focus in the atria
c. It is not life threatening
d. It is an irregular heartbeat

66) Which of the following occurs when an electrical impulse passes through a passage other than the AV node and is characterized by a rhythm of up to 250 BPM?
a. AV reentry tachycardia
b. Asystole
c. Sinus tachycardia
d. Atrial fibrillation

67) Which of the following has P waves that are often hidden by the QRS complex?
a. Sinus bradycardia
b. Atrial bradycardia
c. AV reentry tachycardia
d. Sinus reentry tachycardia

68) The following is an example of

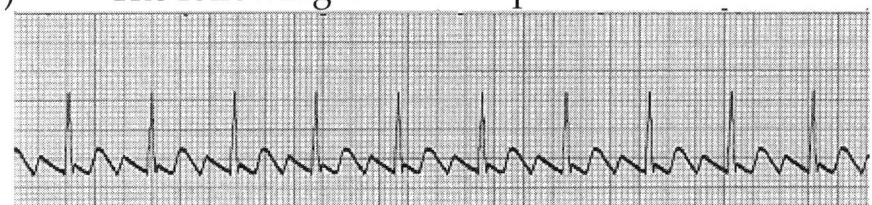

a. AV reentry bradycardia
b. Atrial flutter
c. Ventricular flutter
d. Asystole

69) Which of the following could possible cause atrial flutter?
a. Pulmonary embolism
b. hemodynamic instability
c. Mural thrombi
d. All of the above

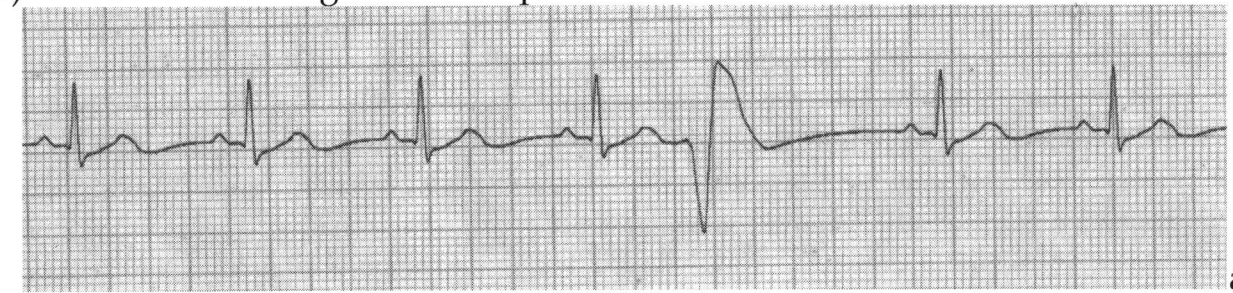

70) The following is an example of

a. Atrial fibrillation
b. Premature ventricular complex
c. Sinoatrial complex
d. Sinoatrial delay

71) Atrial fibrillation is caused by:
a. Multiple irritable sites all over the atria firing at more than 350 BPM
b. Multiple irritable sites all over the ventricle firing at more than 300 BPM
c. Ventricular failure
d. Atrial failure

72) The following is an example of

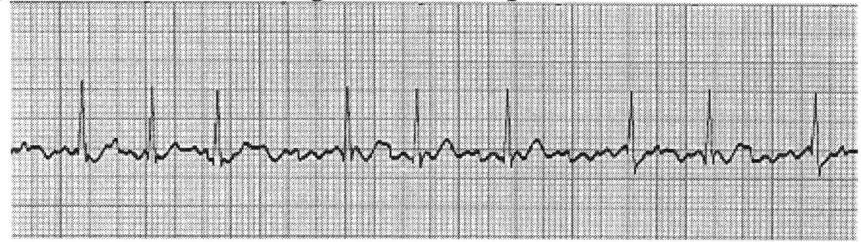

a. Atrial fibrillation
b. Ventricular fibrillation
c. AV node fibrillation
d. Stroke

73) Which of the following is characterized by no identifiable P waves with fibrillatory F waves seen in all leads?
a. Asystole
b. Sinoatrial fibrillation
c. Atrial fibrillation
d. Ventricular fibrillation

74) Which of the following is true about premature ventricular complexes?
a. They do not show up on an EKG reading
b. They arise from irritable sites in the atria
c. The QRS complex is typically less than 0.12
d. They may appear in the same shape or in different shapes

75) Which of the following could cause a premature ventricular complex?
a. Increased catecholamines
b. Decreased blood pressure
c. Increased ventricular activity
d. Decreased heart rate

76) What is the term used for 3 or more PVC's in a row at a rate of over 100 BPM for more than 30 seconds?
a. Sinus tachycardia
b. Ventricular tachycardia
c. Sinoatrial bradycardia
d. None of the above

77) Which of the following is false about ventricular fibrillation?
   a. It is not life threatening
   b. It is caused by quivering of the ventricles
   c. The rhythm is chaotic
   d. It is characterized by waves that vary in shape and size

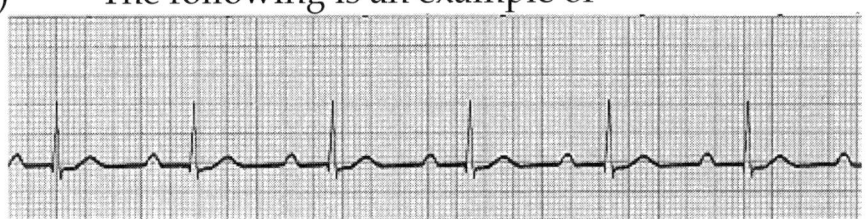

78) The following is an example of

   a. Asystole
   b. First degree heart block type I
   c. Normal sinus rhythm
   d. Sinus bradycardia

79) The following is an example of

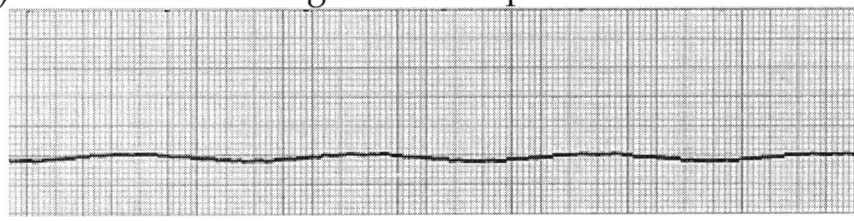

   a. Asystole
   b. First degree heart block type I
   c. Normal sinus rhythm
   d. Sinus bradycardia

80) Type II second degree AV block:
   a. Conducted P waves are normal and PR intervals are normal
   b. Conducted PR waves are normal with unreliable QRS intervals
   c. Conducted P waves have constant PR interval, but there are non-conducted P waves
   d. None of the above

Section Three

81) Which of the following is not a sign of stroke?
   a. Confusion
   b. Atrial fibrillation
   c. Trouble walking
   d. Clear speech

82) Which of the following is one of the three necessary ways to test for stroke outside of the hospital?
   a. Check for facial droop
   b. Check for arm drift
   c. Check for abnormal speech
   d. All of the above

83) A sign of facial droop is:
   a. A crooked smile or impairment on one side
   b. An even smile with even movement
   c. Wrinkles
   d. All of the above

84) An example of arm drift is:
   a. Both arms moving the same
   b. One arm missing
   c. One arm drifting lower than the other when attempting to hold them out
   d. One hand not moving

85) An example of abnormal speech is:
   a. Slurred words
   b. Wrong words from a phrase
   c. Absent words from a phrase
   d. All of the above

86) When should you call EMS during BLS?
   a. After starting compressions

b. After defibrillation
c. Before beginning the ABCD's
d. None of the above

87) When managing respiratory arrest you should:
a. Maintain at least 75% oxygen saturation and airway patency
b. Maintain at least 90% oxygen saturation and airway patency
c. Maintain at least 50% oxygen saturation and airway patency
d. Maintain at least 80% oxygen saturation and airway patency

88) If the patient is expected to have head trauma you should:
a. Avoid giving the patient oxygen
b. Tilt the head back and lift the chin
c. Use the jaw thrust to open the airway
d. Tilt the head forward and open the mouth

89) A patient is semi-conscious, but needs intervention for breathing. Which of the following is the best piece of equipment to use on this patient?
a. Nasopharyngeal airway
b. Oropharyngeal airway
c. Defibrillator
d. None of the above

90) The patient has a great deal of mucous in his/her mouth and is known to have a respiratory ailment that increases mucous. Which of the following should be done to clear out the airway?
a. Defibrillation
b. Suctioning
c. Rescue breaths
d. Chest compressions

91) When a patient is ventilated:
a. Perform CPR in the same way as you would with an unventilated patient
b. Stop resuscitation efforts because ventilation often causes spontaneous breathing
c. Ventilate once every 30 seconds
d. Ventilate once every 5 to 6 seconds

92) Which of the following is a sign of ACS?
   a. Chest discomfort
   b. Shortness of breath
   c. Discomfort in the shoulders and back
   d. All of the above

93) Which of the following is a contraindication of chewing aspirin?
   a. A headache
   b. A recent GI bleed
   c. Blurred vision
   d. A leg cramp

94) Which of the following is a contraindication of nitroglycerine and morphine?
   a. Hypertension
   b. A GI bleed
   c. Hypotension
   d. Blurred vision

95) Which of the following reduces the risk of mortality in STEMI patients?
   a. Reperfusion therapy within the first hour
   b. Blood clotting agents within the first hour
   c. Defibrillation
   d. All of the above

96) Which of the following is an alternative to fibrinoltic therapy in STEMI patients?
   a. ACI
   b. PMN
   c. PCI
   d. CPI

97) Fibrinolytic therapy is not recommended in STEMI patients:
   a. After one hour of symptom onset
   b. After three hours of symptom onset
   c. After six hours of symptom onset
   d. After twelve house of symptom onset

98) What does STEMI stand for?
   a. ST-segment enunciation in mitral infarction
   b. ST-segment elevation in myocardial infarction
   c. ST-segment elevation in mitral ischemia
   d. ST-segment enunciation in myocardial ischemia

99) When should IV nitroglycerin be administered?
   a. When there is pulmonary edema and hypertension
   b. When there is chest discomfort that is not responsive to SL nitroglycerin
   c. When there is chest discomfort that is not responsive to morphine
   d. All of the above

100) Ischemic stroke:
   a. Occurs in 50% of strokes and is a result of hypoxia
   b. Occurs in 80% of strokes and is a result of septicemia
   c. Occurs in 85% of strokes and is a result of a blocked artery in the brain
   d. Occurs in 90% of strokes and is a result of tachycardia

101) Which of the following is false about strokes?
   a. They are easily identified on an ECG
   b. The symptoms vary from patient to patient
   c. They affect the brain
   d. They may only affect one side of the body

102) Which of the following are signs of stroke?
   a. Severe headache
   b. Numbness on one side of the body
   c. Confusion
   d. All of the above

103) Which of the following is one of the three necessary ways to test for stroke outside of the hospital?
   a. Check for facial droop
   b. Check for arm drift
   c. Check for abnormal speech
   d. All of the above

104) When testing for arm droop you should ask the patient to:
   a. Open eyes and relax both arms at the side

b. Close eyes and hold left arm forward palm up
   c. Open eyes and hold right arm forward palm down
   d. Close eyes and extend both arms palms up

105) You respond to a patient who thinks she is having a stroke. She is forty and has obvious signs of asymmetry as well as facial droop. Her speech is slurred. Which of the following is true?
   a. She probably drunk
   b. She is probably faking
   c. She should be treated like she is having a stroke
   d. You should start CPR

106) You respond to a patient whose family member believes he is having a stroke. His speech is slurred. He is thirty years old. He has symmetry and no facial droop. He has a glucose reading of 50. You should:
   a. Treat the patient as if he is having a stroke
   b. Treat the blood sugar issues
   c. Tell him to call back later
   d. Start CPR

107) You arrive at a respiratory arrest scene. The scene is safe. You should:
   a. Begin compressions
   b. Check patient response and activate EMS
   c. Defibrillate
   d. Intubate

108) If bag-mask ventilation is adequate you should:
   a. Continue with ACLS
   b. Implement an advanced airway system
   c. Stop all rescue efforts
   d. Intubate

109) Which of the following reduces the risk of mortality in STEMI patients?
   a. Reperfusion therapy within the first hour
   b. Blood clotting agents within the first hour
   c. Defibrillation
   d. All of the above

110) Which of the following is true about the NPA?
   a. It is inserted over the tongue
   b. It is J shaped
   c. It is inserted through the nostril along the nasal floor
   d. All of the above

111) Which of the following devices could cause damage to the airway if the wrong size is used?
   a. The bag-mask
   b. The OPA
   c. The Catheter
   d. All of the above

112) Which of the following should be rotate 180 degrees as it approaches the pharynx?
   a. The OPA
   b. The NPA
   c. The catheter
   d. The NBC

113) Acute myocardial infarction and acute angina are both part of a spectrum of diseases called?
   a. Acute ventricular syndrome
   b. Acute atrial syndrome
   c. Acute coronary syndrome
   d. None of the above

114) Acute coronary syndrome begins with:
   a. Irregular heartbeats
   b. Plaque buildup
   c. Irregular myocardial contraction
   d. Stroke

115) When is aspirin contraindicated?
   a. When the patient has just eaten
   b. If there is an allergy
   c. If the patient is elderly
   d. If the patient is consciuos

116) If a patient started having chest pains 13 hours ago and is still having chest pain:
   a. The patient can take a clot-busting agent
   b. The patient should take a clotting agent
   c. You no longer need to worry
   d. Any of the above

117) Which of the following is the most important form of PCI?
   a. Clotting agent
   b. Aspirin
   c. Angioplasty
   d. All of the above

118) Which of the following can cause gastritis?
   a. An incorrectly sized OPA
   b. An incorrectly sized NPA
   c. A heart attack
   d. A stroke

119) A patient is unconscious and needs advanced airway support. Which would be the best option for this patient?
   a. Bag-mask
   b. NPA
   c. OPA
   d. Any of the above

120) NSTEMI is a symptom of:
   a. A partially occluded thrombus in the heart
   b. Ventricular tachycardia
   c. Clear veins and arteries
   d. None of the above

Section Four

121) Which of the following is true about strokes?
   a. The symptoms are uniform throughout the event
   b. The symptoms get worse if left untreated
   c. The symptoms go away if ignored

d. Strokes are not life-threatening

122) An elderly person that you have been caring for suddenly is complaining of headaches and has had several personality changes over the past few days. You have noticed that he seems confused from time to time. This could be explained by:
a. Myocardial infarction
b. Getting old
c. Stroke
d. Tachycardia

123) A myocardial infarction can be caused by:
a. Plaque buildup in the blood vessels of the heart
b. Blockage of the blood vessels in the brain
c. A tumor
d. Blockage of the vessels in the abdomen

124) A myocardial infarction can cause:
a. Increased blood flow to the body
b. Increased oxygenation of the heart muscles
c. Death of the tissues in the heart
d. Death of the tissues in the brain

125) A patient has dizziness, fainting, and chest pains. You should:
a. Treat the patient as if he is having a heart attack
b. Treat the patient as if he is having a stroke
c. Treat the patient as if he has the flu
d. Observe the patient

126) Silent ischemia occurs in __% of heart attacks.
a. 10%
b. 8%
c. 25%
d. 19%

127) Early treatment of a heart attack involves:
a. Reducing the severity of the pain
b. Reducing the severity of the damage to the heart
c. Reducing the severity of the damage to the brain

d. All of the above

128) The purpose of nitroglycerin is to:
   a. Thin the blood
   b. Increase heart rate
   c. Decrease the heart's workload
   d. all of the above

129) When is a clot-busting drug most effective?
   a. During the first hour
   b. During the second day
   c. During the first week
   d. During the first three to four hours

130) Which drug prevents ventricular flutter and ventricular tachycardia?
   a. Metroprolol
   b. Lidocaine
   c. Aspirin
   d. Tylenol

131) A patient is complaining of indigestion. He also appears to be sweating and short of breath. Which of the following statements is true?
   a. He could be having a heart attack
   b. It is important to rule out a heart attack
   d. All of the above

132) Which of the following is true about Isoproterenol (Isuprel)?
   a. It produces an increased heart rate
   b. It increases myocardial contractility
   c. It has been replaced with newer and more effective medications
   d. All of the above

133) Which of the following is the drug of choice for suppression of ventricular ectopy?
   a. Metroprolol
   b. Aspirin
   c. Lidocaine
   d. Epinephrine

134) Which of the following is successful 90% of the time in the treatment of PVST?
   a. Lidocaine
   b. Epinephrine
   c. Verapamil
   d. Digitalis

135) When starting dopamine you should:
   a. Use highest prescribed dose available
   b. Use the lowest possible dose that causes results
   c. Use the amount suggested on the label
   d. None

136) Beta-blockers may cause:
   a. Congestive heart failure
   b. Headaches
   c. Itching
   d. All of the above

137) Excessive doses of lidocaine can cause:
   a. Congestive heart failure
   b. Sleepiness
   c. Confusion
   d. Neurological changes

138) When administering Verapamil you should:
   a. Monitor blood pressure
   b. Monitor consciousness
   c. Monitor pulse
   d. Monitor oxygen saturation

139) If a patient suspects he is having a heart attack:
   a. Chewing aspirin may reduce heart damage
   b. Chewing Tylenol may reduce heart attack
   c. Taking Ibuprofen may fix the problem
   d. Any of the above medications may work

140) Which of the following statements is true?
   a. During a heart attack symptoms will always present themselves
   b. During a heart attack symptoms will make it clear that a heart attack is happening
   c. During a heart attack the person will always clutch his chest and fall to the ground
   d. During a heart attack the symptoms will range from mild to severe

141) Who should receive Oxygen?
   a. Only children
   b. Only the elderly
   c. All patients who enter the hospital
   d. All patients with chest pain that may be due to cardiac ischemia

142) Who should receive Epinephrine?
   a. Patients with low blood pressure
   b. Patients with atrial tachycardia
   c. Patients in cardiac arrest
   d. All patients

143) Who should receive Oxygen?
   a. Patients with chest pain due to cardiac ischemia
   b. Patients with chest pain and suspected hypoxia
   c. Patients with chest pains and cardiopulmonary arrest
   d. All of the above

144) Who should be given Dopamine?
   a. Patients with hypotension in the absence of hypovolemia
   b. Patients with hypertension in the absence of hypovolemia
   c. All patients
   d. Patients with chest pain

145) Which of the following is a Beta blocker?
   a. Propranolol
   b. Metoprolol
   c. Atenolol

d. All of the above

146) What symptoms do Beta blockers prevent?
   a. Congestive heart failure
   b. Ventricular ectopy
   c. Atrial fibrillation
   d. Bronchospasms

147) Which drug prevents ventricular flutter and ventricular tachycardia?
   a. Metroprolol
   b. Lidocaine
   c. Aspirin
   d. Tylenol

148) Which drug is best for treatment of paroxysmal supraventricular tachycardia?
   a. Dopamine
   b. Lidocaine
   c. Verapamil
   d. Digitalis

149) Which drug increases the force of the cardiac contractions?
   a. Verapamil
   b. Metroprolol
   c. Aspirin
   d. Digitalis

150) Which of the following is a common side-effect of nitroglycerin?
   a. Fever
   b. Trembling
   c. Headaches
   d. Addiction

151) A stroke where a blood clot forms in a vessel in the brain is:
   a. Embolism stroke
   b. Thrombotic stroke
   c. Cystic stroke
   d. Neural stroke

152) A stroke that occurs when a piece of a blood clot breaks off from another area of the body and is transported to the brain is called:
a. Embolism stroke
b. Thrombotic stroke
c. Cystic stroke
d. Neural stroke

153) Headaches are a symptom of:
a. Bleeding from the stroke
b. Pressure from the blocked blood vessels
c. Side effects from medication
d. All of the above

154) What is a myocardial infarction?
a. Normal blood flow in the heart
b. A lack of blood to the heart tissues
c. A fast heart beat
d. Heart skipping a beat

155) A heart attack is often thought to be_____during the early stages.
a. A stroke
b. Asthma
c. Heartburn
d. Influenza

156) Which of the following is a useful way of treating heart attacks?
a. Chest compressions
b. The Heimlich maneuver
c. Percutaneous coronary intervention
d. Rescue breaths

157) Which of the following is a useful way of treating a heart attack?
a. Chest compressions
b. Blood thinning medications
c. Exercise
d. Sleep

158) Which of the following statements is false?
   a. Some heart attacks do not present any pain symptoms
   b. All heart attacks should be treated as soon as possible
   c. Pain from heart attacks is often mistaken for indigestion
   d. A heart attack deprives the heart of oxygen

159) Which of the following is a false statement?
   a. Stroke victims often show signs of confusion
   b. Stroke victims can survive by getting rest instead of medical treatment
   c. The severity of the stroke depends on the location of the stroke in the brain
   d. Early detection is key to minimizing the damage from the stroke

160) Which of the following statements is true?
   a. It is always obvious when a stroke begins to happen
   b. Symptoms of stroke may occur off and on in the early stages
   c. Only elderly people suffer from strokes
   d. Strokes are not terribly dangerous

Answers

1) B
2) C
3) A
4) D
5) B
6) D
7) C
8) A
9) B
10) D
11) D
12) A
13) B
14) C
15) D
16) B

17) C
18) B
19) A
20) D
21) C
22) D
23) A
24) D
25) A
26) D
27) D
28) A
29) B
30) C
31) A
32) B
33) C
34) D
35) A
36) B
37) B
38) A
39) B
40) C
41) B
42) D
43) C
44) A
45) C
46) C
47) A
48) C
49) D
50) D
51) C
52) B
53) D
54) C
55) A

56) B
57) B
58) A
59) D
60) C
61) C
62) B
63) D
64) D
65) C
66) A
67) C
68) B
69) D
70) B
71) A
72) A
73) C
74) D
75) A
76) B
77) A
78) B
79) A
80) C
81) D
82) D
83) A
84) C
85) D
86) C
87) B
88) C
89) A
90) B
91) D
92) D
93) B
94) C

95) A
96) C
97) D
98) B
99) D
100) C
101) A
102) D
103) D
104) D
105) C
106) B
107) B
108) A
109) A
110) C
111) B
112) A
113) C
114) B
115) B
116) A
117) C
118) B
119) C
120) A
121) B
122) C
123) A
124) C
125) A
126) C
127) B
128) C
129) D
130) B
131) D
132) D
133) C

134) C
135) B
136) A
137) D
138) A
139) A
140) D
141) D
142) C
143) D
144) A
145) D
146) C
147) B
148) C
149) D
150) C
151) B
152) A
153) A
154) B
155) C
156) C
157) B
158) A
159) B
160) B

OTHER TITLES FROM THE SAME AUTHOR:

1. Work At Home Jobs For Nurses & Other Healthcare Professionals
2. Nurses' Romance Series
3. BLS for Healthcare Providers Student Manual
4. Patient Care Technician Exam Review Questions: PCT Test Prep
5. IV Therapy & Blood Withdrawal Review Questions
6. EKG Technician Study guide
7. EKG Test Prep
8. Phlebotomy Test Prep Vol 1, 2, & 3
9. The Home Health Aide Textbook
10. How to make a million in nursing

And Many More Books

Visit www.janejohn-nwankwo.com

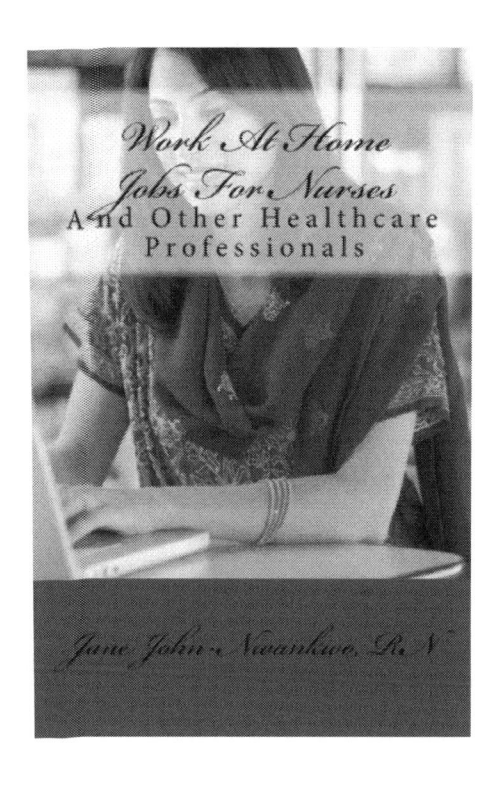

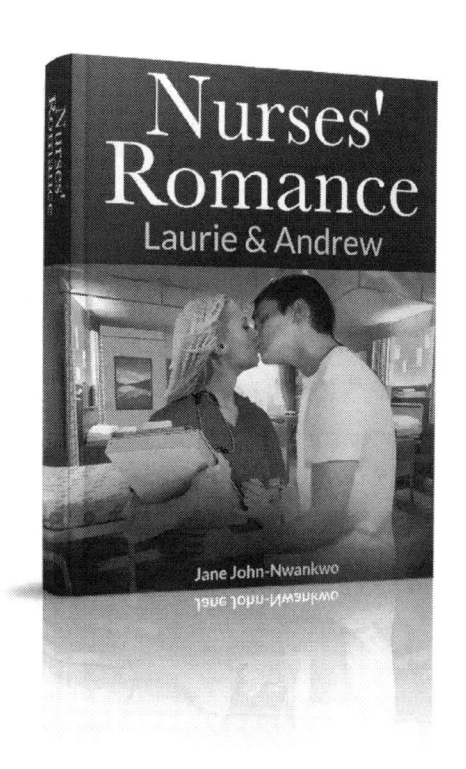

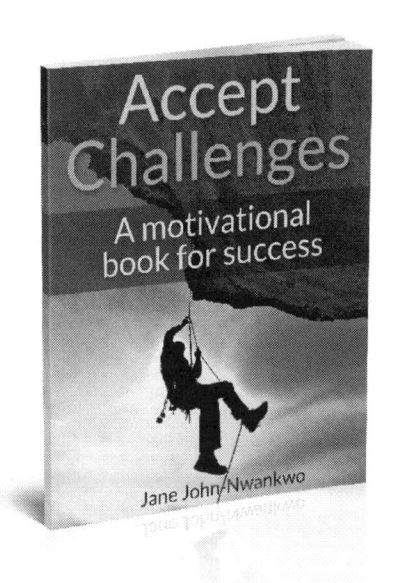

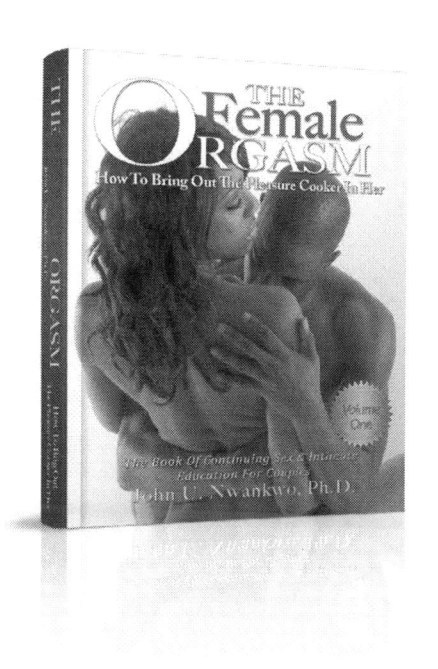

Purchase at www.amazon.com

Made in the USA
Middletown, DE
23 March 2018